The Low-Sugar Cookbook

The Low-Sugar Cookbook

Delicious and Nutritious Recipes to Lose Weight,
Fight Fatigue and Protect Your Health

NICOLA GRAIMES

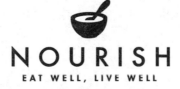

NOURISH

EAT WELL, LIVE WELL

The Low-Sugar Cookbook
Nicola Graimes

This edition first published in the UK and USA in 2014 by
Nourish, an imprint of Watkins Publishing Limited
PO Box 883, Oxford, OX1 9PL, UK

Email: enquiries@nourishbooks.com

A member of Osprey Group

For enquiries in the USA and Canada:
Osprey Publishing
PO Box 3985, New York, NY 10185-3985
Tel: (001) 212 753 4402
Email: info@ospreypublishing.com

Copyright © Watkins Publishing Limited 2010, 2014
Text copyright © Nicola Graimes 2010, 2014

Recipes taken from *Quick & Easy Low-Sugar Recipes*, published by DBP in 2010.

The right of Nicola Graimes to be identified as the Author of this text has been asserted
in accordance with the Copyright, Designs and Patents Act of 1988.

Managing Editor: Sarah Epton
Typeset by: Gail Jones

A CIP record for this book is available from the British Library

ISBN: 978-1-84899-975-6

10 9 8 7 6 5 4 3 2 1

Typeset in Nexus Serif
Printed and bound by CPI Group (UK) Ltd, Croydon, CR0 4YY

Publisher's Note: While every care has been taken in compiling the recipes for this book,
Watkins Publishing Limited, or any other persons who have been involved in working
on this publication, cannot accept responsibility for any errors or omissions, inadvertent
or not, that may be found in the recipes or text, nor for any problems that may arise as a
result of preparing one of these recipes. If you are pregnant or breastfeeding or have any
special dietary requirements or medical conditions, it is advisable to consult a medical
professional before following any of the recipes contained in this book.

nourishbooks.com

Contents

FOOD WARNING SYMBOLS

If you or a member of your family is vegetarian or has an allergy to or intolerance of nuts, eggs, seeds, gluten, wheat or dairy products, you will find these symbols, which accompany each recipe, invaluable. They indicate the presence of a particular ingredient, and any added sugar is also identified.

(V) vegetarian

(⊘) contains nuts

(O) contains eggs

(⊘) contains seeds

(⊘) contains gluten

(⊘) contains wheat

(⊟) contains dairy

(⊞) contains added sugar

In addition, the menu plans on pages 224–227 give ideas for a week's worth of meals for wheat- and gluten-free, vegetarian, vegan and nut-free diets.

NOTES ON THE RECIPES

Please note that metric and imperial measurements are given for the recipes. Follow one set of measures only, not a mixture, as they are not interchangeable.

• 1 tsp = 5ml   1 tbsp = 15ml   1 cup = 250ml

Unless otherwise stated:

• Use medium/large eggs
• Use medium fruit and vegetables
• Use fresh herbs

Introduction

For many years, saturated fat has been the bad boy of the food world, but sugar has now replaced it at the top of the "foods-to-avoid" list. This is because there is growing concern among health experts that, while we've been told for many years to reduce the amount of fat we eat, and a low-fat diet is the key to good health and weight management, people in the developed world are generally becoming fatter and unhealthier. Rates of obesity – and the subsequent health problems that go with it – are at worrying levels and predicted to rise steeply in the future.

The amount of sugar we eat has spiralled upwards – and often without us fully realizing. The root of the problem seems to be the large quantities of soft sugary drinks and processed foods many people are consuming. Laden with sugar, particularly the cheap, subsidized high-fructose corn syrup, these foods are blamed for the rise in obesity, Type 2 diabetes, fatty liver syndrome, cancer and heart disease. And then there are the so-called "healthy" low-fat products; it turns out that, despite the health claims, many of these foods are loaded with sugar, which is often used as a replacement for fat.

Many believe – me included – it's time to take control of what we eat and get back in the kitchen. By preparing and cooking your own meals you are in charge of which ingredients go into them.

You will have noticed that this book is a "reduced-sugar" cookbook, rather than a "no-sugar" cookbook. It is not a diet book either. Instead it's a collection of over 100 delicious and nutritious recipes – both sweet and savoury – all of which have been developed with as little sugar or refined carbohydrates as taste and feasibility allows. The aim of the book is to show you that eating low-sugar foods doesn't mean you're condemned to a dull, tasteless diet; it aims to inspire you to cook delicious, quick and easy, low-sugar meals for all the family. I may be chastised for saying this, but, for me, cakes and puddings are two of life's joys. This book isn't about cutting out those treats completely. But it makes sense from a health – body and mind – point of view to be conscious and aware of how much sugar we consume on a regular basis. Sugar is incredibly pervasive in our diets and it's very easy for the amount we eat to get out of control without even realizing. It makes a great deal of sense to view puddings and cakes as treats and not necessarily something we have to eat every day.

For me, a low-sugar way of eating is firstly about cutting out highly processed foods and sugary drinks; choosing complex carbohydrates, or carbs (see page 10), in preference to refined carbs; eating good-quality proteins and fats; and spoiling myself with the occasional cake, cookie or treat, but not every day (though I will admit to a daily habit of a couple of squares of high-cocoa dark/baking chocolate); and also not giving up fruit but being mindful of not over-indulging on the super-sugary ones, such as dried fruit and bananas.

I really hope this doesn't sound self-righteous, but I've managed to retrain my palate over the years to enjoy foods with a reduced sugar content, so cutting down on the amount I add to cakes, cookies and puddings, stopping taking sugar with tea and coffee, avoiding icing on cakes and biscuits, and cutting out high-sugar jams and the like. I'm by no means perfect, but this approach suits me. And I hope by trying some of the recipes in this book you'll agree that you can make great-tasting dishes, both sweet and savoury, that are low in sugar and full of nutritious, wholesome ingredients.

WHAT IS SUGAR?

Before you can reduce the amount of sugar you eat, you need to get to know a bit more about "the enemy" and its various forms. Sugar is a sweet-tasting simple carbohydrate and comes in numerous guises, the most common being sucrose (regular sugar, which is typically half glucose and half fructose); fructose (found in fruit); and lactose (found in milk). The sugar found in fruit and milk is naturally occurring and also provides vitamins and minerals. Added sugars are typically from sugar cane, beet and corn. While these provide plenty of calories, they contain little or nothing in the way of nutrients and are referred to as "empty calories".

Generally, sugars have names that end in "ose", so alongside the most common types mentioned above there are dextrose, maltose and galactose, but just to confuse matters there are also molasses, cane sugar, coconut sugar, syrups, honey and fruit juice concentrates (see Read the Label, page 21).

CHOOSING THE RIGHT CARBOHYDRATES

Reducing the amount of sugar you eat is only part of the story, because it's also relevant to consider your intake of carbohydrate foods as a whole. If you are looking for sustained amounts of energy and to control any fluctuations in blood-sugar levels – and aren't we all – it's important to eat the right carbs.

Generally classified as complex and simple, depending on their structure, carbohydrates are obtained from beans, pulses, grains, pasta, rice, vegetables, fruit and milk. Despite some people advocating a severely restricted carbohydrate diet, this food group plays an important role in the body and is its main source of energy. When digested, most types of carbohydrate are broken down into simple sugars, otherwise known as glucose. Glucose supplies energy – and in some cells and tissues, such as the brain, it is the vital source of energy. The body works hard to keep glucose levels in check, through the release by the pancreas of the hormone insulin. Carbohydrates also help in the processing of fat and are needed for building the non-essential amino acids that the body requires to create proteins.

Types of Carbohydrate

- Unrefined simple sugars found in fruit and starchy vegetables (fructose) and in milk (lactose)

- Refined simple sugars, such as white and brown sugar (sucrose)

- Unrefined starches or complex carbohydrates, found in whole grains, brown rice, quinoa, barley, lentils, pulses and root vegetables

- Refined starches found in white pasta, white flour, white bread, white rice, cakes, cookies and processed breakfast cereals

---

The more unrefined the carbohydrate you eat, the better it is for your health. A diet based on whole grains, brown pasta, beans, pulses, oats, quinoa and barley is preferable because it will provide the body with bundles of energy, as well as a range of beneficial nutrients and fibre. Fibre is important since it encourages the slow release of sugars (glucose) into the bloodstream, which has a stabilizing effect on blood-sugar levels. Don't forget fruit and vegetables too, which play a vital part in a nutritionally balanced diet.

In contrast, refined versions of carbohydrate, such as white flour and white rice, have had much of their nutritional value and fibre removed during processing. These foods – along with their sugary counterparts – cause extreme fluctuations in blood-sugar levels, leading to unwanted peaks and troughs. These adversely affect energy levels and can lead to mood swings, irritability and hunger pangs.

GLYCAEMIC INDEX OR GLYCAEMIC LOAD?

Some health experts believe that the glycaemic index (GI) is the preferred indicator to the best carbohydrates since it classifies foods according to

how quickly they release sugar (glucose) into the bloodstream. High
GI foods cause a rapid rise in blood-sugar levels, to which the body
responds by releasing insulin. On the other hand, low GI foods release
glucose more steadily over several hours, so less insulin is required.
All carbohydrate foods have a ranking of zero to 100. There are some
anomalies in the GI rating system though, since the method of processing,
the ripeness of a fruit, whether the food is cooked, as well as the fat,
protein and fibre content, will all influence the rating and may not have
been taken into account.

A further criticism of the glycaemic index is that some foods with a
high GI may not necessarily contain a high level of carbohydrate, since
the scale was formulated on a standard weight of carbohydrate (50g/1¾oz)
and not based on an individual serving. For example, in the case of carrots,
which contain only 7 per cent carbs, you would have to consume an
unrealistic quantity to reach 50g/1¾oz carbohydrate content.

Consequently, the glycaemic load (GL) was created to take into account
the amount of carbohydrate present in a single serving, and it is seen as a
more balanced and relevant indicator of sugar content.

HOW MUCH SUGAR SHOULD WE EAT?

There is no actual dietary requirement for sugar as there is for
carbohydrates. A recent survey in the UK revealed that the average British
adult consumes about 700g/1lb 9oz sugar a week – that's around 140
teaspoons. Disturbingly, health experts say our bodies are equipped to
deal with less than half of that amount. The World Health Organization
(WHO) agrees and in 2006 recommended that "added" sugars (those added
to foods, rather than found intrinsically) should make up no more than 10
per cent of our total daily calorie intake.

This means that women should limit their daily consumption of added
sugars to around 50g/1¾oz (10 teaspoons) and men to around 70g/2½oz

(14 teaspoons). Yet the typical diet of many people in the West is double this amount on a daily basis. To put this into perspective, if you eat 3 chocolate biscuits and drink 2 cups of coffee, each sweetened with 2 teaspoons of sugar, you quickly reach the maximum recommended daily level. Drink a can of cola and you are adding a further 9 teaspoons of sugar. Health experts advise that we avoid foods with more than 2 teaspoons of added sugar per serving.

To calculate the number of teaspoons of sugar in a food, divide the number of grams by 5 (a teaspoon is actually 4.9g, although it's easier to calculate if the figure is rounded up to 5).

According to UK government guidelines, a food is high in sugar if it contains more than 15g/½oz sugar per 100g/3½oz, while a low-sugar food contains 5g/½oz or less per 100g/3½oz. Anything in between has a medium sugar content.

The World Health Organization is considering cutting, by up to half, the amount of sugar it recommends, following reviews of the scientific evidence link with obesity. Already, many health experts say added sugar intake should be as low as 30g/1oz (6 teaspoons) for women and 40g/1½oz (8 teaspoons) for men.

Maximum recommended daily carbohydrate/sugar intake for adults:

WOMEN:	MEN:
Cals/day: 1,900	**Cals/day:** 2,550
Total carbs/day: 255g/9oz	**Total carbs/day:** 340g/12oz
Added sugar/day: 50g/1¾oz	**Added sugar/day:** 70g/2½oz

SUGAR AND HEALTH

It is now widely accepted that overall consumption of sugar is currently way above recommended levels, and experts worldwide believe that this is having serious repercussions on our health. The list of related health problems is staggering. A high sugar intake has been linked to an increased risk of heart disease, cancer, diabetes, obesity, dental decay, depression, chronic fatigue, sugar dependence, syndrome X (insulin resistance) and mood swings, and that's just for starters.

Evidence suggests that children are particularly vulnerable to the adverse side effects of a high-sugar diet, namely obesity, behavioural difficulties, mood swings, dental problems, fatigue and poor concentration. A recent UK government report shows that almost 1 in 10 children starting primary school is obese, and unfortunately this problem is not restricted to a single country. Poor diet can also influence a child's health later in life, increasing the risk of developing diabetes, cancer and heart disease.

SUGAR AND OBESITY

According to recent studies, there are now 1 billion people who are overweight worldwide, and 300 million are clinically obese. In the UK, a 2012 survey found that a quarter of all adults in England are obese and this figure is rising. Furthermore, the number of cases of Type 2 diabetes is increasing at a disturbing rate.

While all types of sugar can have a negative impact on our health if eaten to excess, fructose, in particular high-fructose corn syrup (HFCS), sometimes known simply as corn syrup, is currently at the forefront of criticism. Nutritionally void, HFCS has become the cornerstone of processed foods and is often used in unacceptable quantities in both sweet and savoury items – this goes to explain why HFCS has been attributed to the increasing incidence of obesity and diabetes in the USA. (An additional concern is that many processed foods tend to be high in fat, additives and salt.) Made from corn, which is cheap and subsidised in the USA, HFCS comprises 2 types of sugar: fructose and glucose.

Fructose has traditionally enjoyed a healthy reputation, mainly because it does not raise blood-sugar levels, but health experts now believe it to be the cause of many health problems, including weight gain, because of the way it is processed, digested and absorbed in the body. Put simply, most sugars we eat are made up of chains of glucose. When glucose enters the body, it releases the hormone insulin to help regulate it. Fructose, unlike glucose, does not stimulate insulin production and is processed in the liver. When large amounts of fructose enter the liver, the liver has difficulty in processing it fast enough, so any surplus is turned into fat and cholesterol and enters the bloodstream as triglycerides, which is a risk factor for heart disease. This can eventually lead to insulin resistance and non-alcoholic fatty liver disease.

There is also evidence to suggest that fructose circumvents the normal appetite-regulating hormones in the body, encouraging over-eating, which may go some way in explaining the link with weight gain, especially around the abdomen, and subsequently Type 2 diabetes.

Naturally occurring fructose found in fruit does not appear to have the same biological effect in the body as the fructose found in corn syrup, and this is likely because the former is a complex combination of fibre, vitamins, minerals, phytonutrients and antioxidants, while the latter has no nutritional value at all. So eating a moderate amount of fructose from fruit and vegetables is not a bad thing.

SUGAR AND THE HEART

In the past, the focus has been on saturated fat as being the major risk factor in heart disease, but new research shows that sugar plays a greater role than was originally thought. A recent study, which looked at sugar intake and the health of men and women over a 15-year period, showed that the more added sugar a person consumed, the greater the risk of dying from heart disease. There are a number of possibilities: sugar has been shown to increase blood pressure, it increases unhealthy blood fats such as triglycerides, and it increases "bad" LDL cholesterol and depletes "good" HDL cholesterol.

Another problem lies in the effect that sugar and refined carbohydrates, such as white bread, pasta and rice, have on blood-sugar levels. Research shows that they cause a spike in blood sugar and the greater the rise, the more the risk increases of developing cardiovascular disease in the long term. Even transient rises in blood sugar may be a risk factor. Peaks in blood-sugar levels also encourage free radical damage, affect circulation and increase the likelihood of blood clots. This may explain why diabetics have an increased risk of heart disease.

A diet high in fructose (see left) presents additional problems for the health of the heart. A 2009 study from the University of California showed that a high-fructose diet encouraged the build up of fat around the major organs, including the heart, liver and digestive system.

SUGAR AND DIABETES

Until recently, it was believed that there was no direct evidence that sugar causes diabetes. There has always been an indirect link, however, as the risk of developing Type 2 diabetes is related to obesity – and a diet high in sugar leads to weight gain. But a new US study identifies a possible link, separately from obesity. The findings suggest that the longer a country is exposed to what is termed "excess sugar", the higher the incidence of diabetes among the population. When sugar became less available, then rates of diabetes fell, too.

While this study is not conclusive, it can't be denied that the number of people diagnosed with Type 2 diabetes has jumped more than 60 per cent in the UK in just 10 years, and newly released figures suggest that an increase in obesity is fuelling the soaring rates. In the 6-year period 1997–2003, the number of new cases soared 74 per cent, and they rose

63 per cent across the entire decade. In addition, the number of cases of Type 1 diabetes, which usually develops in childhood, and Type 2 diabetes, which is linked to obesity, rose dramatically between 1996 and 2005. These findings suggest that the number of diabetes sufferers in the UK is increasing faster than in the USA, where prevalence of the disease is one of the highest in the world.

Furthermore, consistently elevated levels of insulin in the body, usually the result of eating something sugary, can be detrimental in the long term. Our cells become less responsive to the presence of insulin, so our bodies produce more and more to compensate. Eventually the cells stop responding at all and this leads to Type 2 diabetes.

Diet is the cornerstone of controlling Type 2 diabetes and it's imperative to keep blood-sugar levels within the desired range and keep within a desired weight. It is not believed necessary to cut sugar out completely or even severely restrict carbohydrate intake; however, it is important to eat a healthy, balanced diet that is low in sugar and saturated fat and high in fibre.

SUGAR AND CANCER

The World Health Organization (WHO) believes we have underestimated the influence of diet as a cause of cancer, which is set to rise dramatically in years to come. Diets high in sugar, particularly sugary drinks, processed food and alcohol have come under fire, along with the more obvious lifestyle choices of smoking and lack of exercise.

SUGAR AND AGEING

Evidence suggests that sugar can have an adverse effect on the skin, causing wrinkles and accelerating the ageing process. To blame is a natural process known as glycation, whereby sugar, or more accurately glucose, in the bloodstream attaches to proteins to form harmful new molecules called "advanced glycation end-products" (or, rather appropriately, AGEs).

Most vulnerable to damage are collagen and elastin, which are responsible for keeping the skin firm and elastic. Glycation increases with the more sugar you eat, but the following steps can help to keep your sugar intake in check and, in turn, look after your skin.

- Cut your intake of added sugar to 10 per cent of calories (see page 12).
- Watch out for hidden sugars that lurk in all manner of processed foods (see page 22).
- Increase your intake of antioxidant-rich foods such as fruit, vegetables, nuts and seeds, especially those rich in vitamins C and E as well as beta carotene (converted to vitamin A in the body). The glycation process damages antioxidants through the creation of harmful free radicals, but you can redress the balance through eating foods that are high in antioxidants.
- Vitamins B1 and B6 are known to be AGE inhibitors. These nutrients are found in fruit, vegetables, whole grains, eggs, meat, poultry, seafood, pulses and nuts.

WAYS TO CUT DOWN ON SUGAR
There are many ways you can reduce the amount of sugar in your diet and the following suggestions will help you on your way.

- Try to eat regular meals, starting with a nutritious, low-sugar breakfast. Eating regularly will provide you with sustained amounts of energy throughout the day and stabilize blood-sugar levels, curbing any desire to binge on sugary foods. Studies have found that those who skip breakfast have a tendency to fill up on high-sugar, high-fat snacks mid-morning.

- Replace high-sugar breakfast cereals with porridge (oat, quinoa, millet), home-made muesli or whole grain cereals with no added sugar.

Sugar Cravings

Is sugar addictive? There is a definite correlation between a diet high in sugar and an overall nutritionally deficient diet. This is because sugar tends to displace healthy food in a diet and has been found to encourage overeating. Sugar can leave us feeling uplifted because it prompts the body to release the "happy" hormone serotonin and this makes us feel good. However, what goes up has to come down and this may explain why we get sugar cravings and a desire for a quick sugary fix. Cravings often coincide with a lull in energy or a drop in blood-sugar levels, particularly mid-afternoon. The reason why this often occurs in the afternoon is that the body may have experienced a temporary high in blood sugar after lunch, especially after eating something like a sandwich or other refined carbohydrate food.

One way to avoid such cravings is to keep blood-sugar levels steady by eating regular meals/snacks based on foods such as unrefined carbohydrates, combined with protein foods and "good" fats. These types of foods produce a more sustained effect on blood-sugar levels, because they are broken down more slowly in the body and avoid undesirable peaks and troughs.

Added to this, research shows that our bodies aren't able to tell when we've had enough of certain types of sugar, such as fructose. Foods and drinks sweetened with fructose do not trigger the same sense of satiety as other foods with similar calories, leading to over-indulgence and cravings. Interestingly, glucose was found to be more satisfying.

A lack of sleep and tiredness can also lead to binges on sugary foods as the body and mind crave an energy fix.

- Try to make sure meals are made up of a combination of good-quality protein, unrefined carbohydrates, good fats and plenty of vegetables. Choose foods that are low in the glycaemic load (see page 10), as these will have less impact on blood-sugar levels.

- Whenever possible, try to avoid processed foods – and that includes savoury items, too. Shockingly, 80 per cent of processed food in the USA contains added sugar. (See Foods with Added Sugar, page 22.) By avoiding ready-meals, packaged desserts and the like, and making your own meals, you are in control of the ingredients you use and that includes avoiding unwanted sugar, additives, colourings and flavourings.

- A healthy snack can stop blood-sugar levels dropping too low and avoid the desire for a sugary fix. On pages 72 to 78, there are recipes for snacks – or, alternatively, a handful of unsalted nuts, humous with vegetable sticks, kale chips, half an avocado or low-fat cheese with apple wedges or oatcakes all make healthy options.

- Get into the habit of reading labels (see page 21). Steer clear of any food with sugar (and that includes fructose, glucose, syrups, corn syrup, fruit concentrates and the rest) listed in the first three ingredients.

- Cut out fruit-flavoured drinks (most contain insignificant amounts of fruit and therefore little in the way of goodness because the fibre has been removed along with many of the nutrients, which is also true of juice drinks and juices made from concentrates), sodas and other fizzy sweetened drinks, including most sports drinks, which tend to be high in fructose. Sugar in liquid form enters the bloodstream rapidly, causing a severe spike in blood-sugar levels. There is also growing evidence that these drinks are linked to Type 2 diabetes and weight gain, and since they do not satiate the appetite it's easy to overindulge. Drinks sweetened with artificial sweeteners fare little better, only encouraging a sweet tooth; worse still, they have been linked to stomach problems and cancer when consumed in excess. Great alternatives are water flavoured with a squeeze of fresh lemon, lime or slices of cucumber, along with herb teas and fizzy water.

- Although a source of vitamins, minerals and enzymes, fresh fruit juice loses much of its fibre content, which means the natural sugars enter the bloodstream quickly. It's best to dilute fruit juices with water and avoid drinking them on an empty stomach. Vegetables are a preferred option in fresh juices, especially green, leafy ones, or eat the whole fruit or vegetable instead. Blended smoothies made with the whole fruit, almond milk and flavoured with cinnamon and vanilla extract retain both the fibre as well as the beneficial nutrients.

- Fruit plays an important part of a healthy, balanced diet, providing plenty of vitamins, minerals, phytonutrients and antioxidants. Bear in mind that some fruits contain more natural sugars than others: top of the list are dried fruit, bananas, mango, grapes and cherries, while lower down the scale are berries, melon, peaches and nectarines. Fresh is best, but if buying canned fruit, look for fruit in natural juice rather than in syrup.

- Make cakes, biscuits, cookies and muffins an occasional treat to enjoy, rather than an everyday part of your diet. By cutting down on the amount of sugar you eat on a daily basis, you'll find that in time you'll desire it less as well as prefer foods that are less sweet.

- It can be shocking to find out how much sugar is included in ready-made dressings, marinades, ketchups, jams and sauces (sweet and savoury). Try making your own to avoid hidden sugars found in store-bought versions and watch out for low-fat versions, since it is not unusual for sugar to replace the fat.

- Drink alcohol in moderation and avoid drinking on an empty stomach – not only is it high in sugar, it also adversely affects blood-sugar levels.

- Stress can be a major trigger for sugar cravings. One way to control stress is exercise, which also supports blood-sugar control to avoid dips that can lead to cravings and feeling sluggish. Instead of automatically reaching for a chocolate bar when the afternoon slump hits, try taking a brisk 15-minute walk. A recent study showed that those who took an exercise break were less likely to opt for a sugary snack to perk up energy levels.

READ THE LABEL

Understanding food labels can be a minefield, especially when it comes to working out the sugar content. There are generally two figures for carbohydrates: "Total carbohydrates xxg" and "Of which sugars xxg". Look for the second figure, which will give you a more accurate picture of the sugar content – although some food producers conveniently omit this information, especially if the food is high in sugar! It also makes more sense to look at the "per serving" figure, rather than "per 100g".

Additionally, take time to read the ingredients list to check if there are any added sugars. If sugar features in the first 3 listed ingredients, then it's best avoided as you can guarantee the food will be predominantly sugar. Sugar comes under many guises: anything ending in "ose" can usually be assumed a sugar, including dextrose, fructose, glucose, lactose, maltose, saccharose, sucrose and xylose. Just to confuse matters, there are others, including (high-fructose) corn syrup, corn sweetener, corn syrup solids, fruit concentrates, fruit syrup, invert sugars, honey, maltodextrin, maple syrup, molasses, dextrin, cane juice, malt syrup, raw sugar, rice syrup, sorghum, sorghum syrup, treacle, turbinado syrup and hydrolized starch, brown rice syrup, coconut sugar, barley malt syrup, beet sugar, crystalline fructose, palm sugar, agave and raw sugar.

When reading labels, bear in mind that 1g of sugar contains 4 calories so a store-bought (supposedly "healthy") cereal bar with 20g/¾oz of sugar will instantly add 80 calories on top of everything else. One teaspoon of sugar contains 15 calories.

FOODS WITH ADDED SUGAR

Sugar can appear in the most unlikely of places, but it is its presence in savoury foods and supposedly healthy or low-fat products that is most disturbing. Here is a list of foods – some obvious, others less so – to look out for:

BAKED GOODS

Cakes, biscuits, cookies and crackers (sweet and savoury), breads, brioche, crumpets, English muffins, scones, waffles, pancakes, pastries, croissants, pies, tarts, cheesecakes, cereal bars and flapjacks/bar cookies, cake and batter mixes, flavoured rice cakes and oatcakes, breadsticks.

CANNED FOODS

Vegetables, vegetables in sauce, baked beans, pulses, fish/meat in sauce, spaghetti in tomato sauce, ravioli, pie fillings, soups, tomatoes, cooking sauces, fruit in syrup.

CONDIMENTS

Oriental, Far Eastern and Middle Eastern sauces and pastes, soy sauce, barbecue sauce, tomato ketchup, pickles, salad dressings, mustard, mayonnaise, tomato paste, sandwich spreads, pesto, gravy granules, stock cubes, liquid stock, peanut butter.

DAIRY

Natural/flavoured yogurts, yogurt drinks, pro- and prebiotic drinks, mousses, fools, crème caramel, tarts, ice cream, flavoured cheese spreads, cheese snacks.

SNACK FOODS AND DRINKS

Crisps/potato chips, pretzels, cheese biscuits and crackers, flavoured nuts, cocoa powder, malted drinks, fizzy drinks, fruit squashes, flavoured water, cordials, fruit juices and smoothies.

MEAT, FISH AND SEAFOOD

Pâtés, cured meats, sausages, sausage rolls, ready meals, burgers, pies, pizza, flans, breaded fish and meat, processed potato products.

ABOUT THE RECIPES

Many of us choose to follow a reduced-sugar diet for a plethora of reasons, including a reduced risk of Type 2 diabetes and heart disease, to lose weight, or simply a desire to be healthier. The recipes in this book take this into account by sticking to the recommended guidelines that ensure a balanced and varied diet. The easy-to-follow recipes are divided into 6 chapters covering all occasions, from the all-important first meal of the day through to sweet treats. Savoury foods can be surprisingly high in added sugar, particularly canned and bottled foods and sauces, and you'll find specially adapted recipes for healthier, low-sugar alternatives. Special attention has been given to ensuring that you're not overloading on all types of carbs, especially refined ones. So you'll find recipes for Snacks, Light Meals and Dinners that are low in carbohydrates, and if they do feature then it's in the form of brown rice, quinoa, whole grains, legumes and wholemeal spelt pasta.

The book also makes an important distinction between "added" refined sugars and sugars found "naturally" in fruit, vegetables and complex carbohydrates. Sugars found naturally in fruit play a key part in some of the recipes in this book, but special attention has been made to using the whole fruit – skin included – so the fibre is retained. Along with providing sweetness, fruit is also a good source of beneficial vitamins, minerals, phytochemicals and antioxidants. When baking, fruit helps to keep a cake moist and light, which can be lost when you reduce the sugar content. Spices such as nutmeg and cinnamon are also useful for disguising the fact that there is little sugar as well as adding a wonderful aroma and flavour.

NATURAL SUGAR ALTERNATIVES

Where necessary, xylitol or stevia are used, but not to excess. These natural sugar alternatives do not raise blood-sugar levels in the same way as regular sucrose, or have the health implications associated with fructose. Xylitol and stevia enable you to reduce the amount of sugar needed in, say, a cake without compromising on the end result.

Xylitol

Xylitol is a naturally occurring substance that looks and tastes just like sugar and is said to have a number of health benefits, including improving bone density, controlling the growth of candida (an overgrowth of yeast in the body) and reducing tooth decay. It is found in many plants and fruits and is even made in small amounts by the human body. Xylitol is low GI, and has 40 per cent fewer calories than sugar. What makes it valuable in baking is that it can be used in the same way as ordinary sugar (sucrose), but you need to reduce the oven temperature by 25°C/50°F/Gas 1 as cakes do tend to brown more quickly. Do keep in mind that xylitol can have a laxative effect or cause cramping if eaten in large quantities.

Stevia

Stevia has been used in Japan as a sweetener for several decades, but is relatively new in the West. Three hundred times sweeter than regular sugar and with neglible calories, stevia is produced from a tropical plant native to Latin America. It is sold in both granular and liquid forms and only very small amounts are needed. It does have a slightly bitter, aniseedy flavour that some find off-putting so it pays to try different brands; look for pure stevia, most usually found in health food stores, rather than the most widely available products, which contain additional ingredients. Also, while it can be used in baking, because you need only a small amount you have to consider other options for adding substance and moisture to the bake, such as fruit and vegetable purées. Healthwise, studies have shown that stevia has little impact on blood-sugar levels, assists weight loss, helps to regulate blood pressure and improves digestion. If using liquid stevia then 1 or 2 drops is enough in a cup of water, while 1 teaspoon of the powdered variety is the equivalent of 1 cup of sugar. As with xylitol, it's wise to use stevia in modest amounts and only occasionally.

Other Natural Sweeteners

Other forms of natural sweetener are also used in some of the recipes. These are organic brown rice syrup, pure maple syrup, raw honey and lucuma, which, along with adding the desired amount of sweetness, provide a number of health benefits, including vitamins and minerals. *Brown rice syrup* is made by culturing rice with enzymes to break down the starches. It contains soluble complex carbohydrates, maltose and a small amount of glucose and is free from fructose. Both *maple syrup* and *honey* contain some fructose, but in lower amounts than corn syrup, agave syrup or sucrose. Look for pure and raw versions for the best quality. *Lucuma* powder is produced from a sub-tropical fruit of the tree of the same name that is native to South America and is becoming increasingly popular as an alternative sweetener. Its taste, a cross between maple syrup and caramel, is useful for sweetening baked goods, smoothies and desserts. It is a source of complex carbohydrates and fibre, and contains numerous vitamins and minerals. It is low on the glycaemic index and therefore does not have an unsettling affect on blood-sugar levels. Nevertheless, sugar alternatives are still sugar in one form or another, so limit yourself to small amounts and eat occasionally.

Importantly, there's no need to resort to artificial sweeteners such as aspartame, the adverse health effects of which are well documented if consumed in large quantities. In this book, whenever a recipe calls for sugar in one form or another, then you can be sure that it also includes fibre and protein, which both help to slow down the release of glucose into the bloodstream and also curb the impact of any spikes in blood-sugar levels.

There are numerous health benefits to choosing low-sugar foods or, indeed, opting for the wider parameters of a low-sugar diet, but remember that eating some sweet foods in moderate amounts doesn't make you a weak person or necessarily unhealthy. We are programmed to choose sweet foods from an early age. Breast milk is sweet, and in nature sweetness is a sign that a food is safe to eat. The problems linked with sugar have largely occurred with the burgeoning processed food market, and especially when sugar is combined with fat. Consider this, in nature sugar and fats are rarely found in the same foods... so natural is best.

BASIC LOW-SUGAR RECIPES

Store-bought dressings, sauces, relishes, chutneys, jams and spreads can be notoriously high in sugar as well as containing a surprising number of additional ingredients such as fillers and additives. This versatile collection of basic recipes provides sweet and savoury alternatives that are not only lower in sugar than their ready-made counterparts, but are made with fresh ingredients. All these recipes can be stored in the refrigerator in an airtight container.

Tomato Relish

Ditch the ketchup and opt instead for this refreshing, zingy relish that goes well with grilled/broiled meats, fish, poultry, cheese and vegetarian dishes. It's also good spooned over brown rice or wholewheat couscous. It is best served at room temperature.

SERVES 4   PREPARATION 10 **minutes**

4 vine-ripened tomatoes, quartered, deseeded and finely chopped
juice of 1 lime
1 red onion, finely chopped
1 mild green chilli, deseeded and finely chopped
1 small handful mint, finely chopped
salt and freshly ground black pepper

Put all the ingredients in a bowl and stir until well combined.

(V)

Fresh Coconut Chutney

Chutneys, by their very nature, are laden with sugar; this fresh and zingy alternative is great with eggs and cheese dishes, as well as curries or other spicy food.

SERVES 4   PREPARATION **15 minutes**

55g/2oz/scant 1 cup unsweetened desiccated/shredded coconut
juice of 1 lime
1 large handful chopped mint leaves
1 large handful chopped coriander/cilantro leaves
1 medium green chilli, deseeded and finely chopped
salt, to taste

1   Put the coconut in a bowl and stir in the lime juice and 125ml/4fl oz/
    ½ cup water. Set aside for 10 minutes.

2   Stir the herbs and chilli into the coconut mixture and season with salt,
    to taste. Serve at room temperature.

Mint Raita

Use this perfect cooling accompaniment to hot, spicy curries, stews, or tandoori meat and poultry in place of sugar-laden chutneys. It also makes a delicious salad dressing for mixed green leaves, sprouted beans, or grated uncooked courgette/zucchini.

SERVES 4   PREPARATION **10 minutes**

150ml/5fl oz/scant ⅔ cup low-fat plain yogurt
10cm/4in piece cucumber, halved lengthways, deseeded and finely chopped
5 tbsp finely chopped mint
1 tsp fresh lemon juice
½ tsp cumin seeds

1   Put all the ingredients, except the cumin seeds, in a bowl and stir until well combined.

2   Sprinkle the cumin seeds over the top before serving.

Tzatziki

This typical Greek appetizer is made with courgette/zucchini instead of the usual cucumber. It can be served as a dip or as a reviving accompaniment to spicy dishes.

SERVES 4   PREPARATION 10 minutes

1 courgette/zucchini, trimmed and grated
1 small garlic clove, minced
150ml/5fl oz/scant ⅔ cup 2% fat Greek yogurt
juice of ½ lemon
salt and freshly ground black pepper

Put all the ingredients in a bowl and stir until well combined.

Three-nut Butter

*Sugar is an ingredient you would least expect to find in peanut butter,
but it's often included in store-bought versions. By making your own nut
butter, you can ensure it contains only the ingredients you want and no
additives. You can also use whatever combination of nuts you like. This
nut butter can be stored in an airtight container in the refrigerator for up
to 2 weeks.*

MAKES **200g/7oz**   PREPARATION **10 minutes**   COOKING **5 minutes**

50g/1¾oz/scant ½ cup blanched whole almonds
50g/1¾oz/scant ½ cup unsalted cashew nuts
50g/1¾oz/scant ½ cup unsalted peanuts
90ml/3fl oz/generous ⅓ cup coconut oil, melted
sea salt, to taste

1   Toast the nuts in a dry frying pan for 4–5 minutes, turning once.
    If necessary, rub the nuts in a clean tea towel to remove the papery
    brown covering.

2   Transfer the nuts to a food processor or blender and process until
    finely ground. Pour in the oil and blend to a coarse paste, adding a
    little warm water if the mixture if very thick. Season with salt, to taste.

(V)

Reduced-sugar Strawberry Jam

I did debate whether to include this recipe and you may question my decision to go with it, but for me this book is all about reducing the amount of sugar you eat, rather than cutting it out altogether. This makes an intensely fresh and fruity, high-fruit, no-added-sugar spread that can be used as a filling for cakes, a topping for cheesecakes, or stirred into coconut yogurt or porridge/oatmeal. Store in an airtight container in the refrigerator for up to 1 week.

MAKES **300g/10½oz/2 cups**   PREPARATION **5 minutes**   COOKING **20 minutes**

300g/10½oz/2 cups strawberries, hulled and halved
1 tbsp xylitol or a few drops of liquid stevia, to taste
1 tbsp fresh lemon juice

1   Wash the strawberries under cold running water and leave to drain. Put them in a saucepan with the xylitol and lemon juice and cook over a medium-low heat, stirring occasionally, for 5 minutes until starting to break down.

2   Remove the pan from the heat and mash the fruit with the back of a fork, then return to the heat and cook, half-covered, for 10–15 minutes until reduced and thickened – it should have a chunky syrupy texture. Set aside to cool before using.

Almond Milk

While it's now relatively easy to find nut milk in food stores, much of it is sweetened and it's so much nicer (and so easy) to make at home. This makes a rich milk, and by reducing the amount of added water you could also make an alternative to cream. Almond milk, or you could use cashews, is lactose-free (a form of sugar found in cow's milk), so will suit those who are lactose intolerant.

MAKES **1l/35fl oz/4 cups**   PREPARATION **15 minutes, plus soaking**

200g/7oz/scant 1⅓ cups shelled blanched almonds

1   Leave the almonds to soak in plenty of water overnight (or for up to 2 days), then drain and rinse under cold running water.

2   Put the soaked almonds in a blender with 1l/35fl oz/4 cups (preferably filtered) water and blend on high for 2 minutes, or until the nuts are broken down into a fine meal and the water is creamy white.

3   Strain the almonds through a nut milk bag or muslin-lined sieve, reserving the strained milky liquid in a bowl. Gather up the sides of the bag, or the muslin in the sieve, and squeeze over the bowl to extract as much liquid as possible. Pour the milk into a lidded container. It will keep in the fridge for up to 3 days. The nut meal left in the bag or muslin can be added to muesli or granola.

BREAKFASTS & BRUNCHES

It may be a cliché, but breakfast is certainly the most important meal of the day, replenishing vital nutrients and energy depleted overnight. Recent research suggests that children who eat a decent breakfast perform better at school, and no doubt the same can be said of most adults at work.

However, what you eat is equally as important as when. Eating, for example, a high-sugar cereal for breakfast leads to a temporary surge in blood-glucose levels, which will be promptly followed by a mid-morning slump and subsequent hunger pangs and lull in energy levels. The following recipes enable you to ditch sugary refined cereals in favour of more sustaining and nutritious Cinnamon Porridge with Pear, Blueberry & Almond Bircher Muesli or On-the-day Muesli, which is a healthy combination of nuts, fruits, seeds and oats and can literally be thrown together depending on what you have to hand.

Research also shows that people who avoid breakfast tend to binge on unhealthy, high-sugar, high-fat snacks mid-morning, so if eating first thing is not really you then why not try the Vanilla Shake or Tomato & Almond Booster?

For a more substantial savoury option, turn to the recipes for Baked Eggs & Spinach, Sardines & Tomato on Toast, or Cottage Cheese Pancakes to keep you going through to lunchtime.

Avocado & Coconut Smoothie

This is a cross between a smoothie and a soup, so could be called a "smoopie". It makes a nutritious, hydrating, summery breakfast and is surprisingly filling. The hint of green chilli gives a definite lift, which may be most welcome at the start of the day!

SERVES 2   PREPARATION **10 minutes**

1 small ripe avocado, halved, stoned, peeled and chopped

1 small cucumber, deseeded and sliced

1 yellow pepper, deseeded and chopped

2 spring onions/scallions, chopped

2 tbsp chopped coriander/cilantro leaves

1 medium-hot green chilli, deseeded and sliced

300ml/10½fl oz/scant 1¼ cups unsweetened coconut water

splash of Tabasco

juice of 1 lime

4 ice cubes

1   Put the avocado, cucumber, yellow pepper, spring onions/scallions, coriander, green chilli, coconut water, Tabasco, lime juice and ice cubes in a blender and blend until smooth and creamy.

2   Add a little extra coconut water if the smoothie is too thick. Serve straightaway.

* Health Benefits

Avocados have come under criticism for their high fat content but these healthy fats have been found to boost levels of good HDL cholesterol and protect the body against harmful free radicals. They are also surprisingly rich in protein in a readily digestible form.

Food Facts per Portion
Calories 180kcal • **Total Carbs** 9.3g • **total sugar** 3.2g • **added sugar** 0g

Variation
Smoothies are incredibly versatile and it is well worth experimenting with your own favourite combinations of fruit and vegetables according to what is in season. The beauty of smoothies over juices is that the blended fruit and vegetables retain their beneficial fibre and nutrients that sit just below the skin.

Vanilla Shake

Creamy and sustaining, this protein-rich shake is just the thing to get you going in the morning, but is not too heavy if you're not a big fan of breakfast. Look for good-quality vanilla protein powder, or you could use soya or hemp protein powders instead.

Lucuma powder, from the Peruvian fruit of the same name, is a malty tasting, natural sweetener and a nutritious alternative to regular sugar.

SERVES 2   PREPARATION **10 minutes**

375ml/13fl oz/1½ cups unsweetened coconut milk drink

100ml/3½fl oz/scant ½ cup unsweetened coconut yogurt

1 tbsp vanilla protein powder, or protein powder of choice

2 tsp smooth, sugar-free peanut butter

1 tsp vanilla extract

½ tsp ground cinnamon

½ tsp freshly grated nutmeg

1 tbsp ground flaxseeds

1–2 tsp lucuma powder, to taste

1 Put the coconut drinking milk, yogurt, protein powder, vanilla extract, ground cinnamon, nutmeg, ground flaxseeds and lucuma powder in a blender and blend until smooth.

2 Add extra coconut drinking milk if the smoothie is too thick. Serve straightaway.

* Health Benefits

Peanut butter contains valuable soluble fibre, which helps to slow down the absorption of sugar. Lucuma contains a high concentration of calcium, iron, fibre and vitamin C.

Food Facts per Portion

Calories 260kcal • **Total Carbs** 5.8g • **total sugar** 1.8g • **added sugar** 0g

Tomato & Almond Booster

This savoury breakfast "smoothie" contains a bundle of antioxidants, vitamins and minerals, especially B vitamins, which are essential in converting food to energy. Serve with a boiled egg for an extra protein boost and to keep you fuller for longer.

SERVES 2 PREPARATION **10 minutes, plus soaking**

4 sun-dried tomatoes (not in oil)

40g/1½oz/¼ cup blanched whole almonds

2 tomatoes, deseeded and chopped

1 handful basil leaves

2 handfuls spinach leaves, tough stalks removed

2 tsp ground flaxseeds

few chilli flakes, for sprinkling (optional)

1 Soak the sun-dried tomatoes and almonds in 125ml/4fl oz/½ cup
   just-boiled water for 1 hour, or overnight.

2 Tip the tomatoes, almonds and their soaking water into a blender and
   add the fresh tomatoes, basil, spinach and ground flaxseeds. Pour in
   200ml/7fl oz/scant 1 cup water and blend until smooth (add extra water
   if the smoothie is too thick). Serve sprinkled with chilli flakes, if you
   like. Serve straightaway.

* Health Benefits
*Almonds contain useful amounts of vitamin E and are a good source of
monounsaturated fat, both of which have been found to benefit the health
of the heart.*

Food Facts per Portion
Calories 173kcal • **Total Carbs** 5g • **total sugar** 2.5g • **added sugar** 0g

Fig & Vanilla Breakfast Yogurt

This thick and creamy fruit yogurt is a nourishing and energy-boosting blend of protein, slow-release carbohydrates and beneficial fats, making it an excellent start to the day. Figs may be naturally high in sugar, but they are also rich in fibre and valuable minerals. Scatter the nuts and seeds over the yogurt just before serving for a delicious crunchy topping.

SERVES 4   PREPARATION **5 minutes**   COOKING **17 minutes**

40g/1½oz/¼ cup dried ready-to-eat figs, roughly chopped

½ tsp vanilla extract

300ml/10½fl oz/1¼ cups unsweetened coconut or other dairy-free yogurt

4 tbsp unsalted pistachio nuts, roughly chopped

3 tbsp sunflower seeds, toasted

1 tsp flaxseeds

1 tsp chia seeds (optional)

sprinkling of ground cinnamon

1   Put the figs and 300ml/10½fl oz/1¼ cups water in a medium saucepan. Bring to the boil, then reduce the heat and simmer, covered, for about 15 minutes until the figs are very soft.

2   Mash the cooked figs with the back of a spoon or fork until puréed, then leave to cool slightly.

3   Stir the vanilla extract into the yogurt and divide into 4 tumblers or
    bowls. Add 1 heaped tablespoon of the fig purée to each serving and
    stir in for a swirled effect. Scatter with the pistachio nuts, sunflower
    seeds, flaxseeds, chia seeds, if using, and a sprinkling of cinnamon
    before serving.

Storage

Can be stored in an airtight container in the refrigerator for up to 1 day.
The date purée will keep for up to 5 days in the refrigerator.

* Health Benefits

*Figs make a nutritious natural sweetener, and their high-fibre content
means that the sugars are released steadily into the body, but it is best to
eat dried fruit occasionally and in moderation if following a low-sugar diet.*

Food Facts per Portion

Calories 250kcal • **Total Carbs** 13g • **total sugar** 5.5g • **added sugar** 0g

Variations

Try swapping the figs for dried ready-to-eat apricots (the dark-coloured
unsulphured variety have a wonderful rich toffee flavour). Or try grated
apple or puréed raspberries or strawberries.

In place of the pistachios, try roughly chopped walnuts, Brazils or
pecans. Toasted pumpkin seeds would also work.

Blueberry & Almond Bircher Muesli

Oats, apples and almonds provide fibre and slow-release energy to keep you going through the morning. This particular muesli recipe is largely made the night before serving to allow the oats to soften in the nutritious almond milk, which means it is both quick to prepare, saving you precious time in the morning, and easier to digest.

SERVES 4   PREPARATION **10 minutes, plus soaking**

200g/7oz/2 cups rolled jumbo oats

455ml/16fl oz/scant 2 cups unsweetened almond milk

100ml/3½fl oz/scant ½ cup unsweetened coconut yogurt

1 sweet apple (unpeeled), cored and grated

2 large handfuls blueberries

2 tbsp toasted flaked almonds

freshly grated nutmeg, for sprinkling

1   Put the oats in a mixing bowl and pour the almond milk over. Cover
    with cling film and leave in the refrigerator overnight.

2   Just before serving, stir in the yogurt and grated apple. Spoon into
    4 bowls and top with the blueberries, almonds and a sprinkling of
    nutmeg before serving.

STORAGE

The oat and almond milk mixture can be stored in an airtight container in the
refrigerator for up to 1 day.

* Health Benefits

*Blueberries are high in beneficial antioxidants and they provide significant
amounts of vitamins C and E, which support the immune system.
Especially good for the eyes, blueberries help to protect against macular
degeneration. The soluble fibre found in oats helps to balance blood-sugar
levels, whilst the almonds, yogurt and milk provide valuable amounts of
bone-strengthening calcium.*

Food Facts per Portion

Calories 293kcal • **Total Carbs** 33.5g • **total sugar** 5.3g • **added sugar** 0g

On-the-day Muesli

The beauty of making your own muesli is that you can add your favourite grains, fruit, nuts and seeds, or whatever you have to hand. If strawberries are out of season, use any other berries you like for an antioxidant boost, or try chopped pear or apple.

SERVES 1   PREPARATION **10 minutes**

4 tbsp quinoa flakes or millet flakes

1 tbsp pumpkin seeds

1 tsp hemp seeds

2 Brazil nuts, chopped

2 walnuts, broken into pieces

2 tsp ground flaxseeds

100ml/3½fl oz/scant ½ cup unsweetened almond, hemp or
  coconut milk

4 strawberries, hulled and halved or quartered, or other
  fruit of choice

1 Put the quinoa, pumpkin and hemp seeds, nuts and ground flaxseeds
   in a serving bowl. Add the milk and mix until combined.

2 Top with the strawberries and serve.

STORAGE

The dried muesli mixture can be made in bulk and stored in an airtight
container for up to 1 week.

* Health Benefits

*Pumpkin seeds, walnuts and flaxseeds are a great non-fish source
of healthy omega-3 fatty acids, which benefit the eyes, brain and skin.
Sunflower seeds are also brimming with selenium and vitamin E.*

Food Facts per Portion

Calories 275kcal • **Total Carbs** 12g • **total sugar** 3.2g • **added sugar** 0g

Cinnamon Porridge with Pear

Full of valuable soluble fibre, and a host of essential vitamins and minerals, this dish is both wonderfully comforting and sustaining, whilst the chopped pear adds natural sweetness along with vitamin C and antioxidants.

SERVES 4   PREPARATION **5 minutes**   COOKING **12–17 minutes**

100g/3½oz/scant 1 cup jumbo rolled oats

100g/3½oz/1 cup quinoa flakes

600ml/21fl oz/scant 2½ cups unsweetened almond milk, plus extra
  for pouring (optional)

2 tsp ground cinnamon

1 ripe pear, cored and chopped

16 walnut halves, broken

2 tbsp toasted sunflower seeds

1   Put the oats and quinoa in a saucepan with the milk, ground cinnamon and 800ml/28fl oz/3¼ cups water. Bring to the boil, then reduce the heat and simmer, half-covered, for 10–15 minutes until thickened, stirring frequently.

2   To serve, divide the porridge/oatmeal between 4 bowls, then spoon over the chopped pear. Scatter with the walnut halves and sunflower seeds. Pour a little extra almond milk over, if you like, before serving.

* Health Benefits
Oats are high in soluble fibre, which helps to regulate levels of cholesterol and blood-glucose in the body. Surprisingly, cinnamon also plays an important role in balancing blood-sugar levels, behaving in a similar way to the hormone insulin.

Food Facts per Portion
Calories 348kcal • **Total Carbs** 35.8g • **total sugar** 5.3g • **added sugar** 0g

Variation
Berries, apple or cherries would also make a delicious fruity topping in place of the pear.

Chia Breakfast Pudding

Surprisingly filling and a good source of slow-release energy, the tiny black chia seed has an amazing ability to hold liquid and becomes pudding-like when soaked in almond milk. Top with fresh berries for a simple, nutritious breakfast.

SERVES 2   PREPARATION **5 minutes, plus soaking**

3 tbsp chia seeds

240ml/8fl oz/scant 1 cup unsweetened almond milk

1 tsp ground cinnamon

1 tsp vanilla extract

2 tbsp unsweetened coconut yogurt

20g/¾oz/¼ cup pecan halves, toasted

2 small handfuls raspberries

1   Put the chia seeds in a bowl and pour the almond milk over. Add the cinnamon and vanilla and stir well until combined and all the seeds are submerged in the liquid. Leave to one side for 45 minutes or overnight in the refrigerator if more convenient, until the seeds have swelled and the milk has become gelatinous.

2   Spoon into 2 serving bowls and top with a spoonful of yogurt, the pecans and raspberries. Serve straightaway.

STORAGE

The chia pudding will keep for up to 1 day stored, covered, in the fridge.

* Health Benefits

A good source of omega-3 fatty acids, chia seeds are brimming with soluble fibre, calcium, iron, manganese, phosphorus and antioxidants. They are broken down slowly in the body providing long-term energy and keeping blood-sugar levels steady.

Food Facts per Portion

Calories 168kcal • **Total Carbs** 8.6g • **total sugar** 1.5g • **added sugar** 0g

Ⓥ Ⓞ Ⓐ Ⓥ Ⓐ Ⓐ Ⓐ

Fruity French Toast

This deliciously quick brunch would also make a great dessert. For a change, try swapping the berries for other types of fruit, such as nectarines, peaches or apples.

SERVES 4   PREPARATION **5 minutes**   COOKING **5 minutes**

2 large/extra-large eggs

4 tbsp milk

1 tsp vanilla extract

½ tsp ground cinnamon, plus extra for sprinkling

4 slices soya and linseed bread

20g/¾oz/4 tsp coconut oil or unsalted butter

2 tsp brown rice syrup, maple syrup or raw honey

200g/7oz/1¾ cups mixed berries of your choice, such as blueberries, strawberries, raspberries and blackberries (defrosted if frozen)

90ml/3fl oz/heaped ⅓ cup fromage frais

1   Whisk the eggs, milk, vanilla and cinnamon together in a shallow bowl. Dip both sides of each slice of bread in the egg mixture.

2   Melt the coconut oil in a large, non-stick frying pan. Put the slices of egg-soaked bread in the pan and cook for 2 minutes on each side until golden. (You will probably have to cook the French toast in 2 batches.)

3   Sprinkle the French toast with extra cinnamon and drizzle with the syrup, then serve straightaway with the berries and fromage frais on the side.

* Health Benefits

Berries are little baubles of goodness and are a particularly rich source of antioxidants, including anthocyanins. These potent compounds are said to protect the body against the effect of ageing and improve circulation.

Food Facts per Portion

Calories 230kcal • **Total Carbs** 21.6g • **total sugar** 7.9g • **added sugar** 2.2g

Variation

For a savoury version, stir a handful of freshly grated Parmesan into the egg mixture and serve with the Tomato Relish (see page 28).

Baked Eggs & Spinach

These individual baked eggs can partly be prepared in advance to save time in the morning: follow steps 1–2, then cover the ramekins and chill overnight. Serve with seeded wholemeal toast.

SERVES 4   PREPARATION **10 minutes**   COOKING **5 minutes**

500g/1lb 2oz/5½ cups young leaf spinach, tough stalks removed,
   rinsed well
3 tbsp créme fraîche
a little grated nutmeg
4 eggs
55g/2oz/½ cup grated strong Cheddar cheese
salt and freshly ground black pepper

1   Steam the spinach for 2 minutes until wilted. Leave to drain, then
    squeeze out any excess water using your hands.

2 Finely chop the spinach, then mix with the crème fraîche and a little grated nutmeg. Season and spoon the spinach mixture into 4 large ramekins.

3 Preheat the grill/broiler to medium. Break an egg into each ramekin and sprinkle with cheese. Place the ramekins in the grill pan and cook under the preheated grill/broiler for 2–3 minutes until the eggs are just set, then serve straightaway.

STORAGE

The pre-cooked egg mixture can be stored in an airtight container in the refrigerator for up to 1 day, then cooked.

* Health Benefits

Dark green leafy vegetables, such as spinach, are an important source of cancer-fighting antioxidants. Spinach also contains fibre, which can help to reduce harmful levels of LDL cholesterol, so reducing the risk of heart disease and strokes. Its vitamin C content helps the absorption of the iron that is also present.

Food Facts per Portion

Calories 263kcal • **Total Carbs** 2.3g • **total sugar** 2.2g • **added sugar** 0g

Cheese & Tomato Soufflés

If you find the idea of making a soufflé a little off-putting, this version really couldn't be easier, and a hollowed-out tomato makes the perfect container. Serve with seeded wholemeal bread or toast.

SERVES **4**   PREPARATION **20 minutes**   COOKING **20–25 minutes**

4 large beefsteak tomatoes, top 5mm/¼in sliced off

90ml/3fl oz/generous ⅓ cup semi-skimmed milk

2 large garlic cloves, minced

4 eggs, separated

100g/3½oz/¾ cup strong half-fat Cheddar cheese, grated

1 tsp olive oil

salt and freshly ground black pepper

snipped chives, to sprinkle (optional)

1   Preheat the oven to 190°C/375°F/Gas 5. Scoop out the seeds of the tomatoes to make an empty shell. Sprinkle the inside of the tomatoes with salt and place upside-down on a plate. Set aside for 10 minutes, then rinse and pat dry with kitchen paper.

2   Meanwhile, gently heat the milk until just warm, then stir in the garlic
    and egg yolks and three-quarters of the Cheddar. Heat gently, stirring,
    until the cheese has melted and the mixture thickened. Remove from
    the heat and season.

3   Whisk the egg whites in a grease-free bowl until they form stiff peaks.
    Using a metal spoon, stir a spoonful of the whites into the egg yolk
    mixture to slacken it, then fold in the remaining egg whites until they
    are well combined.

4   Grease an ovenproof dish with the olive oil and place the tomatoes
    upright in the dish. Spoon the soufflé mixture into the tomatoes and
    sprinkle with the remaining cheese. Bake in the preheated oven for
    15–20 minutes until the soufflés have risen and are light golden on top.
    Remove from the oven and sprinkle with chives, if using, then serve.

* Health Benefits
*Eggs provide good-quality protein, which is essential for growth and
development, such as the production of hormones, enzymes and antibodies.
Tomatoes are rich in lycopene (which gives the fruit its red colour), which
can protect against cancer.*

___

Food Facts per Portion
Calories 163kcal • **Total Carbs** 3.1g • **total sugar** 3g • **added sugar** 0g

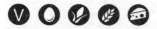

Cottage Cheese Pancakes

These pancakes are given a protein boost thanks to the addition of cottage cheese. They come served with a fresh tomato and basil salad, but if you prefer something warmer, the Home-made Baked Beans (see page 60) go particularly well with them. Serve 1 or 2 pancakes per person, depending on appetite.

SERVES 2–4   PREPARATION **20 minutes**   COOKING **12 minutes**

30g/1oz/¼cup plain/all-purpose wholemeal flour

15g/½oz/1 tbsp unsalted butter, softened, or coconut oil, melted, plus extra for frying

70g/2½oz/heaped ¼ cup cottage cheese

2 eggs

2 tbsp semi-skimmed milk

40g/½oz/scant ½ cup strong Cheddar cheese, grated

½ tsp fresh lemon juice

4 vine-ripened tomatoes, sliced

1 small handful basil leaves

salt and freshly ground black pepper

1 Sift the flour (adding any bran left in the sieve) into a blender. Add the butter, cottage cheese, eggs and milk and whizz to make a batter. Season and leave to rest for 15 minutes.

2 Melt a little butter in a heavy-based frying pan over a medium heat. Pour a quarter of the batter into the pan and swirl the pan until the batter coats the base.

3 Cook the pancake for about 2 minutes, then sprinkle a quarter of the Cheddar over one side. Fold the pancake in half and cook for another minute. Remove from the pan and keep warm while you cook the 3 remaining pancakes, adding more butter in between.

4 Squeeze the lemon juice over the tomatoes, season and top with the basil leaves. Serve the pancakes straightaway with the tomato salad.

* Health Benefits
Cheese provides valuable calcium, which maintains healthy bones and teeth. The mineral is also required for nerve and muscle function. However, dairy produce can be high in saturated fat, so using low-fat versions such as cottage cheese is a good idea.

Food Facts per Portion
Calories 189kcal • **Total Carbs** 6.6g • **total sugar** 2.4g • **added sugar** 0g

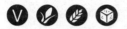

Home-made Baked Beans

Tinned baked beans often contain excessive amounts of sugar and salt, so by making your own you can control which ingredients you use and keep sugar levels to a minimum.

SERVES 4   PREPARATION **5 minutes**   COOKING **25 minutes**

2 tbsp olive oil

1 onion, grated

1 large garlic clove, minced

400g/14oz tin haricot beans in water, drained and rinsed

300ml/10½fl oz/1¼ cups passata (sieved tomatoes)

1 tsp English mustard powder

1 tbsp vegetarian Worcestershire sauce

2 tsp blackstrap molasses

1 tbsp tomato paste

salt and freshly ground black pepper

1   Heat the oil in a saucepan and fry the onion for 8 minutes, stirring occasionally. Add the garlic and cook for another minute or until the onion has softened.

2   Pour in the beans and passata, then add the English mustard powder, Worcestershire sauce, molasses, tomato paste and 4 tablespoons water and stir until combined.

3   Bring to the boil, then reduce the heat and simmer, half-covered, for 10 minutes until the sauce has reduced and thickened. Season to taste, then serve hot.

STORAGE

Can be stored in an airtight container in the refrigerator for up to 3 days, then reheated.

* Health Benefits

Haricot beans are a great source of heart-friendly B vitamins and folate. These help to reduce homocysteine levels, high amounts of which increase the risk of heart disease. The rich, dark blackstrap molasses is a good source of iron, calcium, magnesium, potassium and zinc.

Food Facts per Portion

Calories 150kcal • **Total Carbs** 14.9g • **total sugar** 3.3g • **added sugar** 1g

Salmon Nori Roll

This Japanese-inspired breakfast will fuel the brain and body without loading it with unwanted sugar. Nori sheets make a great alternative to flour-based wraps and conveniently can be kept in the store cupboard for months. Serve with a cup of warming miso soup made simply by stirring a spoonful of paste into a cup of hot water.

SERVES 1   PREPARATION **10 minutes**   COOKING **25 minutes**

1 nori sheet

½ tsp miso paste

70g/2½oz tinned wild pink salmon, drained, skin and bones removed

2.5cm/1in piece cucumber, deseeded and cut into strips

green part of 1 spring onion/scallion, cut into strips

¼ red pepper, deseeded and cut into strips

1 tsp alfalfa sprouts

1 Lightly toast the nori sheet in a large, dry frying pan for 1 minute until starting to turn crisp.

2 Remove the nori from the pan and spread the miso paste down the centre of the sheet. Top with the salmon, cucumber, spring onion/ scallion, red pepper and alfalfa sprouts. Roll up the nori to make a long roll, then cut crossways in half before serving.

STORAGE

Can be stored wrapped in cling film in the refrigerator for up to 1 day.

* Health Benefits

Like other sea vegetables, nori is rich in minerals, including iron, zinc, magnesium and calcium as well as vitamins A, B and K. It is also a good source of iodine, which is essential for thyroid health.

Food Facts per Portion

Calories 185kcal • **Total Carbs** 10.3g • **total sugar** 4.4g • **added sugar** 0g

More-fish-than-rice Kedgeree

This nutritionally balanced, substantial breakfast-cum-brunch provides an energy-giving combination of complex carbohydrates, protein, vitamins and minerals. It would also make a filling main meal served with extra green veg.

SERVES 4   PREPARATION **15 minutes**   COOKING **30–35 minutes**

175g/6oz/scant 1 cup brown basmati rice

2 bay leaves

2 tsp low-salt bouillon powder

55g/2oz/scant ¼ cup red lentils

500g/1lb 2oz undyed smoked haddock fillets

3 tbsp unsalted butter or coconut oil

1 large onion, chopped

2 tsp black mustard seeds

150g/5½oz/1½ cups spinach leaves, tough stalks removed

4½ tsp garam masala

4 green cardamom pods, split

2 tsp ground turmeric

4 hard-boiled eggs

freshly ground black pepper

1   Put the rice in a saucepan and pour in sufficient water to cover it by
    1cm/½in. Add the bay leaves and bring to the boil. Stir in the bouillon
    powder, then reduce the heat to its lowest setting. Cover the pan and
    simmer for 25–30 minutes until the water has been absorbed. Remove
    the pan from the heat and leave to stand, covered, for 5 minutes.

2   Meanwhile, put the lentils in a pan, cover with water and bring to the
    boil. Reduce the heat slightly and simmer, part-covered, for 15 minutes
    or until tender. Drain and leave to one side.

3   Put the fish in a large sauté pan and cover with water. Bring to the boil,
    then reduce the heat and simmer for 3–5 minutes until cooked. Using
    a fish slice, take the fish out of the water (reserving 90ml/3fl oz/⅓ cup),
    remove the skin and any bones and flake the fish into large chunks.

4   Heat half the butter in the cleaned pan and fry the onion for 8 minutes
    until softened, then stir in the mustard seeds for 1 minute. Add the
    spinach and remaining spices and cook for 2 minutes, adding the
    reserved cooking water. Stir in the rice, lentils, haddock and remaining
    butter and turn gently until heated through. Season to taste. Halve the
    eggs and arrange them on top before serving.

STORAGE

The rice can be stored in an airtight container in the refrigerator for up to
2 days, then reheated thoroughly with the onion mixture.

* Health Benefits
    Brown rice provides higher levels of fibre and nutrients, such as vitamins
    B, manganese, magnesium and iron, than white rice.

Food Facts per Portion
Calories 448kcal • **Total Carbs** 36.1g • **total sugar** 2g • **added sugar** 0g

Sardines & Tomato on Toast

Economical and nutritious, tinned fish makes a useful store-cupboard standby. Sardines are often sold whole, even when tinned, so you just need to make sure you remove the spine. Buy the best quality you can afford for maximum taste and nutrition. This dish can be rustled up in a matter of minutes.

SERVES 1   PREPARATION **5 minutes**   COOKING **5 minutes**

1 slice seeded wholemeal bread
2 tinned sardines in olive oil, spine removed
1 vine-ripened tomato, quartered, deseeded and chopped
pinch of crushed dried chillies
4 basil leaves, torn

1   Preheat the grill/broiler to medium-high. Toast the bread on one side.

2   Drain the sardines and mash lightly with a fork, then combine with the chopped tomato.

3   Spoon the sardine mixture on top of the non-toasted side of the bread and sprinkle over the crushed chillies. Grill/broil for 3 minutes under the preheated grill/broiler, scatter with the basil and serve.

* Health Benefits
Our heart, eyes, brain and metabolism all benefit from the omega-3 fatty acids found in oily fish such as sardines.

Food Facts per Portion
Calories 187kcal • **Total Carbs** 13.6g • **total sugar** 2.8g • **added sugar** 0g

Roast Mushrooms with Bacon

This is a definite weekend breakfast-cum-brunch, when you hopefully have a little extra time on your hands for cooking. Don't let that put you off though – it's easy to prepare. You could serve the mushrooms with a slice of seeded wholemeal bread.

SERVES 4   PREPARATION **10 minutes**   COOKING **20 minutes**

4 large portobello mushrooms, stalks removed

2 tbsp olive oil

4 rashers smoked bacon

4 eggs

4 tbsp crème fraîche

salt and freshly ground black pepper

1   Preheat the oven to 200°C/400°F/Gas 6. Place the mushrooms on a piece of foil large enough to make a parcel. Spoon the oil over and season with salt and pepper, to taste. Fold up the foil to encase the mushrooms and place in a baking dish, then cook for 20 minutes until tender.

2 Put the bacon in a separate foil-lined baking tin/pan and cook in the oven with the mushrooms for 20 minutes, turning halfway, or until starting to crisp. Drain on kitchen paper.

3 Meanwhile, poach the eggs. Half-fill a deep frying pan with water and bring almost to boiling point, then turn the heat to low. Swirl the water and break the eggs, one at a time, into the pan. Poach the eggs at a gentle simmer for about 2–3 minutes, then remove using a slotted spoon and drain.

4 Place the mushrooms on serving plates and top with an egg. Place a spoonful of crème fraîche on top of each one. Snip the bacon into pieces and pile on top of the mushrooms. Serve straightaway.

* Health Benefits
  The humble egg is a high-quality protein food, which is rich in B vitamins, especially B12, as well as vitamins A and D along with the minerals iron, choline and phosphorus.

Food Facts per Portion
Calories 341kcal • **Total Carbs** 0.6g • **total sugar** 0.5g • **added sugar** 0g

LIGHT MEALS & SNACKS

Low-sugar diets are not just about reducing the amount of sugar
you eat, but also about cutting your intake of refined carbohydrates
such as crisps, pizza, white bread, white rice, white pasta, breaded
meats and other processed foods. These foods often form the basis
of quick snacks and light meals, yet unfortunately have a similar
negative affect on blood-sugar levels as those foods that are high in
sugar, causing peaks and troughs in energy levels. What's more, many
processed savoury snacks are often high in fat and salt, and, somewhat
surprisingly, may contain added sugar, too.

A couple of nutritious snacks a day will help to sustain energy, aid
concentration and prevent mood swings. Choose from the quick and
easy Soy Nuts & Seeds, Indian-spiced Pulses or Savoury Popcorn.

The light meals, too, are all simple to make – just right when
you don't have a lot of time on your hands – and make the most of
wholegrains, pulses and vegetables, such as the vibrant Warm Greek
Salad of Beans, Basil & Feta, spicy Huevos Rancheros and warming
Vegetable & Chicken Ramen.

(V) ● ● ● ●

Soy Nuts & Seeds

Nuts are brimming with beneficial fats and are also a good source of protein, selenium, iron and fibre. A small handful – about 30g/1oz/scant ¼ cup – is a good snack serving size. Note that some makes of soy sauce contain added sugar, so it's a good idea to check the label before buying, and if you want a wheat- and gluten-free nibble, opt for tamari instead.

SERVES 6   PREPARATION **5 minutes**   COOKING **8–10 minutes**

185g/6½oz/ heaped 1 cup mixed unsalted nuts and seeds such as walnuts,
    Brazils, almonds, cashews, hazelnuts, sunflower seeds and pumpkin seeds
1 tbsp reduced-salt soy sauce (no added sugar)

1   Preheat the oven to 160°C/315°F/Gas 3. Place your chosen selection
    of nuts on a baking tray and roast in the preheated oven for about
    6 minutes.

2   Add the seeds and turn until combined, then roast for another
    2–4 minutes until they smell toasted and are light golden. Keep
    an eye on them because they can burn easily.

3   Remove the nuts and seeds from the oven and transfer them to a bowl.
    Leave to cool slightly, then drizzle the soy sauce over the top and turn
    the nuts and seeds with a spoon until they are coated all over. Serve.

STORAGE

Can be stored in an airtight container for up to 1 week.

* Health Benefits

*Pumpkin seeds are one of the few foods that provide useful amounts
of both healthy omega-3 and omega-6 fats. They are also a good source
of iron – essential for new blood cells – and zinc, which benefits the health
of the skin, hair and nails.*

Food Facts per Portion

Calories 188kcal • **Total Carbs** 3.4g • **total sugar** 1g • **added sugar** 0g

Variation

For spicy nuts and seeds, replace the soy sauce with a spice mix of your
choice – Cajun spices are particularly good. After the nuts and seeds have
been toasted, transfer them to a bowl and sprinkle over 1 tsp Cajun spice
blend. Using a spoon, turn the nuts and seeds until coated.

Indian-spiced Pulses

Chickpeas/garbanzo beans, when roasted, make tasty, crunchy little snacks, and are lower in fat than nuts or crisps and without the unwanted additives. Carotina oil gives a wonderful golden colour to the pulses, but you could use olive oil instead.

SERVES 4   PREPARATION **10 minutes**   COOKING **50 minutes**

400g/14oz tin chickpeas/garbanzo beans in water, drained and rinsed
1 tbsp carotina oil or olive oil
½ tsp low-sodium salt
1½–2 tsp tandoori spice mix

1   Preheat the oven to 170°C/325°F/Gas 3. Line a plate with kitchen paper and tip the chickpeas/garbanzo beans on top. Pat them dry with another sheet of kitchen paper.

2   Tip the pulses into a bowl and add the oil, salt and tandoori spice mix. Stir until the pulses are coated in the spicy oil mix.

3   Spread the pulses over a baking sheet in an even layer and roast in the preheated oven for 50 minutes or until crisp, turning them occasionally. Remove from the oven and leave to cool before serving.

STORAGE

Can be stored in an airtight container for up to 3 days.

* Health Benefits

Chickpeas/garbanzo beans, like other pulses, are high in soluble fibre, stabilize blood-sugar levels and help to lower cholesterol. Their potassium content helps to balance body fluids. Carotina oil is a combination of red palm oil and canola oil and provides more vitamin E (as well as omega-3 and omega-6) than other types of oil.

Food Facts per Portion

Calories 113kcal • **Total Carbs** 11.2g • **total sugar** 0.3g • **added sugar** 0g

Savoury Popcorn

Store-bought popcorn tends to be loaded with sugar, and surprisingly even the savoury versions can be sweetened. Bags of popping corn are readily available in food stores and are much cheaper than the bags of the ready-popped corn available.

SERVES 4   PREPARATION 5 minutes   COOKING 10 minutes

2 tsp coconut oil
100g/3½oz/scant 1 cup popping corn
2 tsp Cajun spice mix
grated zest of 1 lemon
1 tbsp toasted sesame seeds

1   Heat the oil in a medium saucepan with a tight-fitting lid. Add the corn in an even layer, cover with the lid and heat until the corn starts to pop. Shake the pan occasionally and continue to cook until there is no sound of popping.

2   Tip the popcorn into a bowl and spoon the spice mix and lemon zest
over. Sprinkle with the sesame seeds and turn the popcorn until it is
coated in the flavourings and seeds, then serve.

STORAGE

Can be stored in an airtight container for up to 1 day.

* Health Benefits

*Corn provides a good range of nutrients, from B vitamins, vitamins C
and E, folic acid, fibre, essential fatty acids and the minerals magnesium
and phosphorus. The B vitamins are essential for a healthy nervous system,
energy metabolism and brain function.*

Food Facts per Portion

Calories 148kcal • **Total Carbs** 12g • **total sugar** 0.3g • **added sugar** 0g

Variation

For a sweet version, replace the spice mix and lemon zest with a
teaspoonful of brown rice syrup or maple syrup. Pour the syrup over
the popped corn and stir until it is coated.

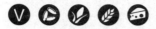

Chickpea Pancakes

These savoury wheat-free pancakes are made with protein-rich gram flour (chickpea flour). Serve them as an accompaniment to curries or as a sustaining snack topped with a spoonful of Fresh Coconut Chutney (see page 29), or dipped into a cooling Mint Raita (see page 30). They would work equally well served with a dollop of Gazpacho Salsa (see page 142) for a more Mediterranean twist.

MAKES 12   PREPARATION **10 minutes, plus standing**   COOKING **16 minutes**

140g/5oz/1¼ cups gram flour (chickpea flour)

½ tsp salt

¼ tsp baking soda

1 tsp nigella seeds

1 tsp garam masala

2 tbsp natural low-fat bio yogurt

groundnut oil, for frying

1   Sift the flour, salt and baking soda into a large mixing bowl. Stir in
    the nigella seeds and garam masala, then make a well in the centre.
    Using a balloon whisk, gradually mix in 200ml/7fl oz/generous ¾ cup
    water, followed by the yogurt, to make a smooth batter. Set aside for
    15 minutes.

2   Heat enough oil to cover the base of a large, heavy-based frying pan
    over a medium heat. Spoon 2 tablespoons of the batter per pancake
    into the pan – you will probably be able to cook 3 or 4 at a time.

3   Cook the pancakes for 2 minutes until light golden, then turn them
    over with a palette knife and cook for a further 2 minutes. Keep
    warm while you cook the remaining pancakes. Serve the pancakes
    straightaway with a topping or dip of your choice.

* Health Benefits
*Along with a beneficial amount of fibre, chickpeas/garbanzo beans provide
useful amounts of heart-protecting magnesium and folate. A deficiency in
these nutrients has been linked to increased incidence of a heart attack.*

Food Facts per Pancake

Calories 54kcal • **Total Carbs** 6.5g • **total sugar** 0.8g • **added sugar** 0g

Omelette "Pizzas"

These "pizzas" couldn't be more simple or quick to make and always go down well with kids. Try adding your favourite toppings – see below for ideas – and serve with vegetable crudités or a mixed salad.

SERVES 4   PREPARATION **10 minutes**   COOKING **20 minutes**

8 eggs
40g/1½oz unsalted butter or coconut oil, for frying
2 tomatoes, deseeded and diced
1 small garlic clove, minced
1 tsp dried oregano
150g/5½oz mozzarella cheese, drained and torn into pieces
16 pitted/stoned black olives, sliced
1–2 tsp extra virgin olive oil
salt and freshly ground black pepper

1   Preheat the grill/broiler to medium-high and line the pan with foil. Mix together the tomato, garlic and oregano.

2   To make the omelettes, crack 2 eggs at a time into a bowl, season with salt and pepper and lightly beat with a fork until combined. Heat 2 teaspoons of butter in a medium-sized, non-stick frying pan with a heatproof handle. When melted, pour in the egg and swirl the pan until the base is coated in the egg. Cook the omelette until just firm.

3   Spoon a quarter of the tomato sauce over the top of the omelette, then sprinkle with the mozzarella. Scatter the olives over the top.

4   Drizzle a little olive oil over the "pizza" and season to taste. Grill/ broil under the preheated grill/broiler for 2–3 minutes or until the mozzarella is just melted. While one omelette is grilling, make the next one and repeat until you have 4 omelette pizzas. Serve straightaway.

* Health Benefits
Make sure olive oil plays a regular part in your diet, since it has been shown to improve the way glucose is absorbed by the cells and also helps to reduce blood pressure.

Food Facts per Portion

Calories 228kcal • **Total Carbs** 0.3g • **total sugar** 0.2g • **added sugar** 0g

Variations
Boost the vegetable content of the "pizzas" by topping them with slices of onion, mushroom or sweet peppers. You could also add cooked chicken, salami, ham or prawns/shrimp.

Tomato & Lentil Soup

Tinned tomato soup contains a surprising amount of added sugar, unlike this home-made version, which features the additional health benefits of lentils. Serve the soup with slices of crusty wholemeal bread.

SERVES 4   PREPARATION **15 minutes**   COOKING **40 minutes**

1 tbsp olive oil

1 large onion, chopped

1 large carrot, peeled and finely chopped

2 celery sticks, finely chopped

250ml/9fl oz/1 cup passata (sieved tomatoes)

750ml/26fl oz/3 cups vegetable bouillon

55g/2oz/¼ cup split red lentils, rinsed

1 bay leaf

1 bouquet garni

salt and freshly ground black pepper

2 tbsp crème fraîche, to serve (optional)

1   Heat the oil in a large, heavy-based saucepan. Add the onion, cover the pan and sauté for 5 minutes until softened and transparent. Add the carrot and celery, cover, and cook for a further 3 minutes, stirring occasionally to prevent the vegetables sticking to the bottom of the pan.

2 Add the passata, bouillon, lentils, bay leaf and bouquet garni and bring to the boil, then reduce the heat and simmer, half-covered, for 30 minutes until the lentils and vegetables are tender and the soup has thickened.

3 Remove the bay leaf and bouquet garni. Using a stick blender, purée the soup until smooth. Season to taste and serve in 4 bowls topped with a spoonful of crème fraîche, if using.

STORAGE

Can be stored in an airtight container in the refrigerator for up to 3 days or the freezer for up to 3 months, then reheated.

* Health Benefits

The lentil is much underused and underrated, but this humble pulse is bursting with nutrients, including B vitamins, which aid the release of energy from foods, and valuable fibre.

Food Facts per Portion

Calories 155kcal • **Total Carbs** 14.3g • **total sugar** 6.2g • **added sugar** 0g

Warm Greek Salad of Beans, Basil & Feta

The cream-coloured butter bean is flavoured with garlic, herbs, feta and lemon to make a warm salad that is packed full of nutrients and robust Mediterranean flavours.

SERVES 4   PREPARATION **10 minutes**   COOKING **5 minutes**

2 tbsp extra-virgin olive oil

3 large garlic cloves, chopped

1 large red pepper, halved, deseeded and diced

800g/1lb 12oz tin butter beans in water, drained and rinsed

2 tsp dried oregano

10 spring onions/scallions, sliced

2 handfuls rocket leaves

juice of 1 lemon

185g/6½oz feta cheese, cubed

1 large handful basil leaves, torn

salt and freshly ground black pepper

1 Heat the oil in a frying pan and fry the garlic and pepper for 1 minute. Add the beans, oregano, spring onions/scallions and rocket and stir gently, then cook for another minute.

2 Stir in the lemon juice and heat through, then season to taste. Divide between 4 plates and top with the feta. Scatter the basil leaves over the top before serving.

STORAGE
Can be stored in an airtight container in the refrigerator for up to 2 days.

* Health Benefits

Tinned pulses make a useful and nutritious addition to the store cupboard. Butter beans provide both types of fibre: soluble (good for the heart) and insoluble (good for the bowel). Basil is said to be good for the digestion, easing constipation.

Food Facts per Portion

Calories 292kcal • **Total Carbs** 16.8g • **total sugar** 1.7g • **added sugar** 0g

Red Quinoa Tabbouleh

Serve this herby salad at room temperature with the slices of freshly chargrilled halloumi placed on top. Halloumi tastes best when served warm straight after cooking.

SERVES 4   PREPARATION **20 minutes**   COOKING **16 minutes**

125g/4½oz/⅔ cup red quinoa

4 vine-ripened tomatoes, deseeded and cut into bite-sized pieces

7 spring onions/scallions, sliced

1 small cucumber, halved, deseeded and diced

35g/1¼oz mint, chopped

35g/1¼oz flat leaf parsley, chopped

juice of 1 lemon

½ tsp crushed dried chillies (optional)

250g/9oz halloumi, sliced

1 tbsp olive oil

salt and freshly ground black pepper

1   Put the quinoa in a saucepan and cover with boiling water. Bring to the boil, then reduce the heat and simmer, covered, for about 10 minutes or until tender. Drain the quinoa, put it in a serving bowl and leave to cool.

2   Add the tomatoes, spring onions/scallions, cucumber, mint and
    parsley. Squeeze in the lemon juice, add the crushed chillies, if
    using, and season well. Stir until combined.

3   Heat a griddle pan or frying pan. Brush the halloumi with the oil
    and cook for 4 minutes or until slightly golden. Divide the tabbouleh
    between 4 plates, top with the halloumi and serve.

STORAGE

The tabbouleh can be stored in an airtight container in the refrigerator for up
to 2 days.

* Health Benefits

*Like golden quinoa, the red variety is a source of complete protein,
providing about the same amount as milk and double that of rice. But
that's not all – quinoa is also gluten-free, low GI and low in fat, a good
source of omega-6 and packed with minerals and B vitamins, so the grain
makes a great contribution to a healthy diet.*

Food Facts per Portion

Calories 185kcal • **Total Carbs** 19.7g • **total sugar** 5.9g • **added sugar** 0g

Avocado & Tomato Bruschetta

This is a simple and delicious combination, but make sure the tomatoes and avocado are nice and ripe for the best flavour. Native to Central America, avocado – sometimes known as a butter pear because of its silky smooth flesh – contains plenty of immune-boosting, anti-ageing vitamin E. For a light lunch or snack, serve the bruschetta with a crisp green salad.

SERVES 2   PREPARATION **7 minutes**   COOKING **3 minutes**

2 thick slices wholemeal soda bread
1 small avocado, halved and pitted/stoned
1 vine-ripened tomato, sliced into rounds
½ tsp balsamic vinegar or fresh lemon juice
½ tsp extra-virgin olive oil
8 large basil leaves
freshly ground black pepper

1   Toast the soda bread on both sides.

2   Meanwhile, scoop the avocado flesh out of its skin with a spoon into a
    bowl, then mash with a fork. Spoon the avocado straight onto the toast
    – there's no need for any butter.

3   Top the avocado with the slices of tomato and drizzle with the balsamic
    vinegar and olive oil. Season with pepper to taste, scatter with the basil
    leaves and serve.

* Health Benefits
  *The body more readily absorbs lycopene, the plant compound found in
  plentiful amounts in tomatoes, when the tomato is cooked, but it is also
  present in raw tomatoes. Lycopene has been found to protect us from
  certain cancers and heart disease.*

Food Facts per Portion
Calories 194kcal • **Total Carbs** 17.5g • **total sugar** 2.4g • **added sugar** 0g

Variation
Ricotta, humous or sliced mozzarella would all make delicious
replacements for the avocado.

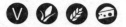

Spicy Tofu Cakes with Dipping Sauce

Tofu really benefits from being combined with more intense flavours, such as herbs and spices. These savoury patties make a light meal served with the dip and a cucumber and onion salad, or, for something a little more substantial, serve with a soba noodle salad.

SERVES 4   PREPARATION **20 minutes, plus chilling**   COOKING **10–14 minutes**

500g/1lb 2oz block firm tofu, drained
2 tbsp curry paste of your choice
2 large garlic cloves, minced
2.5cm/1in piece fresh root ginger, peeled and grated
1 red chilli, deseeded and finely chopped
4 tbsp chopped coriander/cilantro leaves
4 spring onions/scallions, finely chopped
3 tbsp plain/all-purpose wholemeal flour, plus extra for dusting
2 tbsp coconut or olive oil
salt and freshly ground black pepper

For the dipping sauce:
125ml/4fl oz/½ cup natural low-fat bio yogurt
2 tsp fresh lemon juice
2 tbsp chopped mint

1 Pat the tofu dry with kitchen paper, then coarsely grate into a bowl. Add the curry paste, garlic, ginger, chilli, coriander/cilantro and spring onions/scallions. Sift in the flour and a little salt and mix to make a coarse, sticky paste. Cover and refrigerate for 1 hour for the flavours to infuse and to allow the mixture to firm up slightly.

2 Meanwhile, make the dipping sauce by mixing together the yogurt, lemon juice and mint in a bowl, then season to taste.

3 Take large walnut-sized balls of the mixture and, using floured hands, flatten into rounds until you have 12 patties.

4 Heat the oil in a large frying pan and cook the tofu cakes in 2 batches for 4–6 minutes, turning once, until golden. Keep the first batch warm while you cook the second one. Drain on kitchen paper and serve warm with the dipping sauce.

* Health Benefits

Tofu is a curd made from fermented soya milk and is often referred to as a superfood because of its numerous health benefits. Rich in minerals, particularly iron and calcium, it is also low in saturated fat and cholesterol-free. It has been found to help reduce blood pressure and blood cholesterol and the risk of certain cancers.

Food Facts per Portion

Calories 213kcal • **Total Carbs** 12.5g • **total sugar** 1.1g • **added sugar** 0g

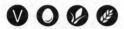

Huevos Rancheros

Traditionally served for breakfast, this Tex-Mex dish makes a simple light meal when served with a large green salad.

SERVES 4   PREPARATION **15 minutes**   COOKING **20–25 minutes**

3 tbsp olive oil

1 large onion, chopped

1 green pepper, halved, deseeded and sliced

1 large garlic clove, chopped

2 tsp ground cumin

½ tsp chilli powder (optional)

2 tsp dried oregano

800g/1lb 12oz/3⅓ cups tinned chopped tomatoes

400g/14oz tin kidney beans in water, drained and rinsed

4 eggs

salt and freshly ground black pepper

1   Heat half of the olive oil in a frying pan. Add the onion and fry gently for 5 minutes, stirring regularly. Add the pepper and cook for 3 minutes, then stir in the garlic and fry for a further 1 minute.

2   Stir in the cumin, chilli powder, if using, oregano, tomatoes and kidney
    beans and bring to the boil, then simmer for 10–15 minutes until
    reduced and thickened. Season to taste.

3   Meanwhile, heat the remaining oil in a large frying pan. Break the eggs
    into the pan and fry until cooked. Divide the tomato and bean sauce
    into 4 bowls and serve topped with a fried egg.

STORAGE

The tomato and bean sauce can be stored in an airtight container in the
refrigerator for up to 3 days or the freezer for up to 3 months, then reheated.

* Health Benefits

*Numerous studies highlight the health attributes of onions and garlic,
particularly their antibacterial, antiviral and antifungal properties. Both
have been found to reduce levels of harmful LDL cholesterol and high blood
pressure as well as raising beneficial HDL cholesterol, reducing the risk of
heart disease and strokes.*

Food Facts per Portion

Calories 256kcal • **Total Carbs** 21.4g • **total sugar** 9.5g • **added sugar** 0g

Asparagus, Courgette & Chive Omelette

This open omelette, topped with delicious spring vegetables, makes an easy light, summery lunch. Serve with a generous mixed green salad and new potatoes, cooked in their skins to retain their maximum nutritional qualities.

SERVES 1   PREPARATION **10 minutes**   COOKING **7–8 minutes**

5 broad/fava bean pods

1 small courgette/zucchini, cut into ribbons with a vegetable peeler

4 asparagus spears, trimmed

1 tsp olive oil

2 eggs, lightly beaten

1 tbsp low-fat garlic soft cheese/farmer's cheese

1 tbsp chopped chives

salt and freshly ground black pepper

1   Shell the broad/fava beans and steam them with the courgette/zucchini and asparagus for about 4 minutes or until the vegetables are tender. Remove the tough outer skin from the beans to reveal the bright green inside.

2   Meanwhile, heat the oil in a medium-sized, non-stick frying pan. Season the eggs and pour them into the pan. Turn the pan until the egg mixture coats the base. Cook for 2–3 minutes, then slip the flat omelette onto a plate.

3   Place a spoonful of soft/farmer's cheese in the middle of the omelette, top with the vegetables, then sprinkle with the chives before serving.

* Health Benefits
Asparagus was used as a medicine long before it was eaten as a food. Rich in vitamin C, asparagus also has diuretic and laxative properties.

Food Facts per Portion
Calories 231kcal • **Total Carbs** 3.7g • **total sugar** 2g • **added sugar** 0g

Mediterranean Salad

This substantial salad makes a nutritious, complete meal in itself. Simply scrub the potatoes rather than peeling them, to help retain the fibre and nutrients found in or just below the skin. Fibre helps to keep blood-sugar levels steady following a meal.

SERVES 4   PREPARATION **15 minutes**   COOKING **10–15 minutes**

200g/7oz new potatoes, scrubbed and halved (if large)
200g/7oz/1½ cups fine green beans, trimmed and halved
2 large handfuls rocket leaves
1 large Little Gem lettuce, shredded
3 large vine-ripened tomatoes, cut into wedges
1 small red onion, thinly sliced into rings
400g/14oz tin chickpeas/garbanzo beans in water, drained
200g/7oz tinned tuna in olive oil, drained and flaked
16 small black olives
4 hard-boiled eggs
salt and freshly ground black pepper

For the dressing:
4 tbsp reduced-fat mayonnaise
1 tsp wholegrain mustard
juice of ½ lemon

1   Cook the potatoes in a saucepan of boiling water for 10–15 minutes until tender, then drain and leave to cool slightly. Meanwhile, steam the green beans until tender and cool under cold running water.

2   Arrange the rocket and Little Gem lettuce on a serving platter, then top with the potatoes, beans, tomatoes, red onion, chickpeas/garbanzo beans, tuna and olives. Halve the eggs, arrange them on top and season.

3   To make the dressing, mix together the mayonnaise with 2 tablespoons water, the mustard and lemon juice, then season. Drizzle the dressing over the salad and serve.

STORAGE

The undressed salad can be stored in an airtight container in the refrigerator for up to 1 day. Add the dressing just before serving.

* Health Benefits

Tuna loses much of its omega-3 content through the canning process, but nevertheless it remains a good source of valuable protein and is low in saturated fat.

Food Facts per Portion

Calories 310kcal • **Total Carbs** 21.8g • **total sugar** 7.2g • **added sugar** 1.3g

Pasta Puttanesca

There is no need to stick to pasta made from refined wheat when there are so many different types to choose from: buckwheat, brown rice and quinoa pasta to name but a few. Spelt is used here, and although it is an ancient wheat variety, it has a lower GL (glycaemic load) than the common wheat we are familiar with.

SERVES 4   PREPARATION **10 minutes**   COOKING **12 minutes**

300g/10½oz wholegrain spelt or quinoa spaghetti

2 tbsp olive oil

2 garlic cloves, finely chopped

6 tinned anchovy fillets

400g/14oz/1⅔ cups tinned cherry tomatoes

200g/7oz tinned chickpeas/garbanzo beans in water, drained and rinsed

1 tsp dried oregano

3 tbsp small black stoned olives

½ tsp crushed dried chillies (optional)

1 heaped tbsp small capers, drained

1 tbsp chopped parsley leaves

salt and freshly ground black pepper

1   Cook the pasta following the instructions on the packet until al dente.
    Meanwhile, heat the oil in a saucepan, add the garlic and fry for
    30 seconds, then add the anchovies and cook, stirring, for 2 minutes
    or until they begin to break up.

2   Stir in the tomatoes, chickpeas/garbanzo beans, oregano, olives, crushed
    chillies, if using, and capers and bring to the boil, then reduce the heat
    and simmer, half-covered, for 5 minutes until beginning to thicken. Stir
    the sauce occasionally to stop it sticking to the base of the pan.

3   Drain the pasta, reserving 3 tablespoons of the cooking water. Return
    the pasta to the pan with the water and sauce and heat through,
    stirring until combined. Season to taste, then sprinkle with parsley
    before serving.

STORAGE

The pasta sauce can be stored in an airtight container in the refrigerator for
3 days, then reheated.

* Health Benefits

*Spelt was one of the first grains to be grown (as long ago as 2500BC) and is
currently experiencing a renewal in popularity. Although spelt is part of the
wheat family, it is generally tolerated by those with a wheat intolerance;
although it should be avoided by people with coeliac disease. It has a
higher nutritional value than wheat, is richer in vitamins B and E and
also contains significant amounts of protein.*

Food Facts per Portion

Calories 366kcal • **Total Carbs** 54.9g • **total sugar** 5.8g • **added sugar** 0g

Chinese Egg & Prawn Rice

This simple meal is a great way of using up leftover brown rice. Brown basmati is best, since the grains remain separate yet fluffy when cooked. Do make sure you reheat the cooked rice thoroughly until it is piping hot.

SERVES 4   PREPARATION **20 minutes**   COOKING **15 minutes**

1 tbsp coconut oil

1 tsp sesame oil

1 large onion, sliced

1 large red pepper, halved, deseeded and sliced

200g/7oz/scant 2 cups choi sum, sliced

2 large garlic cloves, chopped

5cm/2in piece fresh root ginger, peeled and grated

150g/5½oz/1¼ cups frozen petits pois

300g/10½oz cooked and peeled prawns/shrimp

350g/12oz/scant 2 cups cooked cold brown basmati rice

3 tbsp reduced-salt soy sauce (no added sugar)

3 eggs, lightly beaten

1 tbsp sesame seeds, toasted (optional)

1 handful coriander/cilantro leaves, chopped

freshly ground black pepper

1   Heat the coconut and sesame oils in a large wok or frying pan. Add
    the onion and stir-fry for 3 minutes, then toss in the red pepper and
    choi sum and cook, stirring, for 3 minutes.

2   Next add the garlic, ginger and petits pois, then stir-fry for another
    minute. Stir in the prawns/shrimp and rice and heat through,
    stirring continuously.

3   Make a well in the centre of the rice and pour in the soy sauce and
    eggs and draw the rice into the egg mixture, stirring continuously,
    making sure it does not stick to the bottom of the wok.

4   When the egg has cooked, season with pepper, sprinkle with the
    sesame seeds, if using, and scatter with the coriander/cilantro
    before serving.

* Health Benefits
  *The health benefits of ginger have been well documented for centuries,
  but more recent research has shown that ginger reduces blood pressure
  and boosts circulation. Ginger also increases the release of insulin
  secretion and increases the uptake of glucose in fat cells.*

Food Facts per Portion

Calories 345kcal • **Total Carbs** 32.8g • **total sugar** 5.9g • **added sugar** 0g

Spiced Prawns

*Mustard seeds give a warming, nutty flavour and aroma to this light,
quick meal. You can use cooked instead of raw prawns/shrimp: just
simply heat them through for 1–2 minutes at the end. You could serve
the prawns with a warmed wholemeal chapatti.*

SERVES 1   PREPARATION **10 minutes**   COOKING **8 minutes**

1 tbsp sunflower oil

1 red onion, sliced

1 tsp black mustard seeds

1 tsp cumin seeds

½ tsp crushed dried chillies

1 large garlic clove, chopped

1 courgette/zucchini, sliced

8 raw large king prawns/jumbo shrimp, peeled

1 tbsp fresh lemon juice

salt and freshly ground black pepper

steamed spinach, to serve

1   Heat the oil in a wok and stir-fry the onion for 3 minutes. Add the
    spices and garlic and stir-fry for another minute.

2   Add the courgette/zucchini and prawns/shrimp and stir-fry for
    3 minutes or until the prawns/shrimp turn pink and are cooked
    through. Stir in the lemon juice and season to taste, then serve on
    a bed of steamed spinach.

STORAGE

The stir-fry mixture can be stored in an airtight container in the refrigerator
for up to 2 days, then served cold as a spiced prawn/shrimp salad.

* Health Benefits

*Recent data suggests that prawns/shrimp provide reasonable amounts
of omega-3 fatty acids. Like fish, prawns/shrimp are also low in saturated
fat and brimming with protein, B vitamins, zinc, magnesium, selenium
and iodine.*

Food Facts per Portion

Calories 240kcal • **Total Carbs** 23g • **total sugar** 2.9g • **added sugar** 0g

○

Salmon & Onion Frittata

Tinned salmon makes a convenient store-cupboard standby for dishes such as fishcakes, pasta sauces, fish pies or tarts. You could also use tinned tuna or crab for this frittata. Serve with a large green salad.

SERVES **6**   PREPARATION **10 minutes**   COOKING **18 minutes**

420g/15oz tinned wild red salmon, drained
1 tbsp coconut oil
1 large onion, sliced
8 eggs, lightly beaten
salt and freshly ground black pepper

1   Turn the salmon out onto a plate and remove any skin and bones, then flake the fish into large chunks.

2   Heat the oil in a medium frying pan with a heatproof handle, then fry the onion for 8 minutes until softened and slightly golden. Stir in the salmon, retaining the chunks as much as possible. Spread the salmon and onion mixture over the base of the pan in an even layer.

3   Preheat the grill/broiler to medium. Season the eggs and pour them evenly into the pan. Cook for about 5 minutes over a medium-low heat until the base is light golden and set.

4   Place the pan under the preheated grill/broiler and cook the frittata for about 3 minutes until the eggs have just set. Slide out onto a plate and cut into wedges before serving.

STORAGE

Can be wrapped in kitchen foil and stored in the refrigerator for up to 3 days.

* Health Benefits

Long chain omega-3 fatty acids are found in plentiful amounts in salmon and are essential for maintaining a healthy nervous system as well as benefiting the brain, skin and hair.

Food Facts per Portion

Calories 229kcal • **Total Carbs** 3.1g • **total sugar** 2.2g • **added sugar** 0g

Spiced Chicken with Lime Guacamole

Chargrilling or griddling is a great low-fat method of cooking. Serve with a large green salad and Tomato Relish (see page 28).

SERVES 4   PREPARATION 10 minutes, plus marinating   COOKING 35 minutes

2 tbsp fajita spice mix

½ tsp crushed dried chillies

2 tbsp olive oil, plus extra for brushing

600g/1lb 5oz skinless chicken breast, cut into strips

1 large red onion, halved and sliced

1 large red pepper, halved, deseeded and cut into strips

2 courgettes/zucchini, cut into strips

400g/14oz tin black beans in water, drained

For the guacamole:

1 large avocado, halved, pitted/stoned and flesh scooped out

juice of 1 lime, plus a few strips of zest

1 small garlic clove, minced

salt and freshly ground black pepper

1   Mix together the fajita spice mix, crushed chillies and oil in a shallow
    dish. Season with salt and pepper, to taste. Add the chicken and turn to
    coat. Set aside in the refrigerator, covered, for about 1 hour to marinate.

2   To make the guacamole, put the avocado, lime juice and garlic in a
    bowl. Use a fork to mash the avocado to a coarse purée. Season to taste
    and scatter with the lime zest before serving.

3   Heat a griddle pan and remove the chicken from the marinade using
    tongs, then griddle for 8–10 minutes, turning once, until cooked. (You
    will probably have to do this in 2 batches.) Remove from the pan and
    keep warm in a low oven.

4   Put the onion and red pepper in the griddle pan, brushing them with
    a little oil. Cook for 8 minutes, turning once, until slightly blackened,
    then remove and keep warm with the chicken while you griddle the
    courgettes/zucchini for 5 minutes.

5   Meanwhile, tip the beans into a pan, add a splash of water and heat
    through. When the beans are hot, combine them with the onion and
    pepper. Divide the vegetables and beans into 4 plates and top with the
    courgettes/zucchini, chicken and a spoonful of guacamole.

* Health Benefits
*Avocados contain heart-friendly monounsaturated fat. What's more, they
are good source of lutein, which protects the eyes against age-related
degeneration and cataracts. They also have cholesterol-reducing properties,
are a great source of vitamin E and protect against the ageing process.*

Food Facts per Portion
Calories 476kcal • **Total Carbs** 37.8g • **total sugar** 4.9g • **added sugar** 0g

Vegetable & Chicken Ramen

Despite the long list of ingredients, this Japanese-style soup could not be easier to make, and it is light and soothing to eat. Look for soba noodles made with buckwheat flour, which has a lower GL (glycaemic load) than wheat flour.

SERVES 4   PREPARATION **10 minutes**   COOKING **18–20 minutes**

400g/14oz skinless, boneless chicken breasts, sliced into thin strips

olive oil, for brushing

200g/7oz wholegrain soba noodles

4 tbsp brown rice or other miso paste

2 tbsp reduced-salt soy sauce (no added sugar)

5cm/2in piece fresh root ginger, peeled and cut into thin strips

1 large carrot, peeled, halved and cut into matchsticks

6 spring onions/scallions, thinly sliced on the diagonal

1 red pepper, halved, deseeded and cut into thin strips

2 pak choi/bok choy, cut lengthways

1 tsp toasted sesame oil

2 tsp nori flakes

1 small handful coriander/cilantro leaves

1   Preheat the grill/broiler to high and line the grill pan with foil. Place
    the chicken in the grill pan and brush with oil, then grill/broil for
    5–6 minutes on each side until cooked right through.

2   Meanwhile, cook the noodles following the packet instructions, then
    drain and refresh under cold running water and set aside.

3   Put 1 litre/35fl oz/4 cups hot water in a saucepan, add the miso paste
    and stir until dissolved. Add the soy sauce, ginger, carrot, spring
    onions/scallions, red pepper and pak choi/bok choy and bring
    to the boil, then reduce the heat and simmer, uncovered, for about
    3 minutes until the pak choi/bok choy is just tender.

4   Divide the noodles and chicken among 4 shallow bowls and spoon over
    the vegetables and bouillon. Drizzle over the sesame oil, then sprinkle
    with the nori flakes and coriander/cilantro leaves before serving.

STORAGE

Can be stored in an airtight container in the refrigerator for up to 2 days.

* Health Benefits

*The main component of miso is fermented soya beans, although there are
various types available that may also include rice (as used here), barley or
wheat. In some parts of China and Japan, drinking a bowl of miso a day
is a must – ensuring a long and healthy life. It is particularly good for the
digestion and is said to help to eliminate toxins from the body.*

Food Facts per Portion

Calories 423kcal • **Total Carbs** 42.7g • **total sugar** 5g • **added sugar** 0g

Turkey & Apple Salad

Try to eat a rainbow of different-coloured fruits and vegetables each day, since each colour provides a variety of healthy phytochemicals (plant nutrients), vitamins and minerals.

SERVES 4   PREPARATION **15 minutes**   COOKING **5 minutes**

1 apple, quartered, cored and diced (unpeeled)

juice of ½ lemon

400g/14oz tin flageolet beans in water, drained

2 Little Gem lettuces, leaves shredded

2 handfuls rocket leaves

1 carrot, peeled and grated

½ small red cabbage, cored and shredded

2 celery sticks, finely sliced

300g/10½oz cooked skinless turkey breast, sliced

For the dressing:

4 tbsp plain low-fat bio yogurt

3 tbsp reduced-fat mayonnaise

1 tsp extra-virgin olive oil

1 garlic clove, minced

salt and freshly ground black pepper

1 Toss the apple in 2 teaspoons of the lemon juice, which will prevent it from browning.

2 Arrange the beans, Little Gem, rocket, carrot, cabbage, celery and apple in a serving dish.

3 Mix together the ingredients for the dressing with the remaining lemon juice and season well. Arrange the turkey on top of the salad, drizzle the dressing over the top and serve.

STORAGE

The undressed salad can be stored in an airtight container in the refrigerator for up to 1 day. Add the dressing just before serving.

* Health Benefits

Studies show that eating cabbage more than once a week can reduce the likelihood of cancer of the colon in men by up to 65 per cent. Raw cabbage is particularly potent and has antiviral and antibacterial properties.

Food Facts per Portion

Calories 215kcal • **Total Carbs** 15.2g • **total sugar** 5.1g • **added sugar** 0.9g

Bacon, Lentil & Pepper Salad

Tinned lentils keep the preparation of this crunchy salad quick and easy. If you prefer to use dried green or Puy lentils instead, cook them in boiling water until tender.

SERVES 4   PREPARATION 15 minutes   COOKING 7–9 minutes

6 reduced-salt bacon rashers

1 large red pepper, halved, deseeded and diced

2 celery sticks, thinly sliced

6 spring onions/scallions, thinly sliced

2 large handfuls watercress

400g/14oz tin green lentils in water, drained and rinsed

For the dressing:

2 tbsp extra-virgin olive oil

1 tbsp apple cider vinegar

1 tsp Dijon mustard

1 garlic clove, halved

salt and freshly ground black pepper

1   Preheat the grill/broiler to high and line the grill pan with foil. Cook the bacon under the preheated grill/broiler until crisp. Remove and leave to cool slightly, then snip into bite-sized pieces.

2 While the bacon is cooking, put the red pepper, celery, spring onions/ scallions, watercress and green lentils in a serving bowl. Add the bacon to the bowl.

3 Put all the dressing ingredients in a bowl or jug and stir them together using a fork or small whisk. Set aside for 10 minutes to allow the garlic to infuse. Then remove the garlic before pouring.

4 Pour the dressing over the lentil salad, toss together until combined and serve.

STORAGE

The undressed salad can be kept in an airtight container in the refrigerator for up to 3 days. Add the dressing just before serving.

* Health Benefits

Hippocrates is said to have prescribed apple cider vinegar for respiratory problems. In fact, this superfood has been praised for centuries for its numerous health benefits, including improving the symptoms of arthritis, joint pain, acne, candida, digestive disorders and acid reflux. It is even said to aid weight loss. Make sure you buy the unrefined organic variety.

Food Facts per Portion

Calories 220kcal • **Total Carbs** 12.1g • **total sugar** 1.8g • **added sugar** 0g

Beef & Broccoli Stir-Fry

Stir-frying is an excellent method of low-fat cooking. Serve this colourful dish with wholegrain noodles or brown rice. Researchers have found that whole grains may help to reduce the risk of Type 2 diabetes, partly attributed to the presence of magnesium, which promotes healthy blood-sugar control.

SERVES 4   PREPARATION **15 minutes**   COOKING **10 minutes**

350g/12oz long-stem broccoli, stalks diagonally sliced, florets separated

2 tbsp coconut oil

400g/14oz lean beef sirloin, thinly sliced across the grain

1 yellow pepper, halved, deseeded and sliced

1 red pepper, halved, deseeded and sliced

2 pak choi/bok choy, sliced crossways

3 large garlic cloves, sliced

5cm/2in piece fresh root ginger, peeled and cut into thin matchsticks

1 tsp Chinese 5-spice

1 medium-hot red chilli, deseeded and sliced

2–3 tbsp reduced-salt soy sauce (no added sugar)

1 tsp toasted sesame oil

freshly ground black pepper

1   Steam the broccoli for 2 minutes, then refresh for a few seconds under cold running water.

2   Heat the oil in a wok or frying pan until hot. Add half of the beef and stir-fry for 2 minutes until browned and sealed all over. Remove the beef from the wok using a slotted spoon and set aside while you cook the remaining beef.

3   Pour away all but 1 tablespoon of the oil. Put the broccoli, yellow and red peppers, pak choi/bok choy, garlic and ginger into the wok and stir-fry for 2 minutes.

4   Return the beef to the wok and stir, then add the 5-spice, chilli, soy sauce and sesame oil and stir-fry for another minute, adding a splash of water if too dry. Season with pepper and serve.

* Health Benefits
Red meat, such as beef, provides plentiful amounts of iron in a readily absorbable form. Iron is vital for making new red blood cells. Broccoli is a nutritional powerhouse, providing numerous vitamins and minerals and beneficial plant compounds.

Food Facts per Portion
Calories 217kcal • **Total Carbs** 3.9g • **total sugar** 3.3g • **added sugar** 0g

DINNERS

This diverse selection of recipes takes its inspiration from some of the cuisines of the world, including Spanish Chorizo & Bean Stew, Mexican Vegetarian Chilli in Tortilla Baskets, Thai Mussels with Noodles, Moroccan Chicken Pilaf and Beef & Lentil Curry. A nutrient-rich combination of ingredients, such as wholegrains, pulses, lentils and vegetables, features heavily within the recipes in this chapter. These also have a stabilizing influence on blood-sugar levels, keeping hunger pangs at bay for longer. Much is made of low-fat sources of protein, including chicken, seafood, beans and lean cuts of beef, which when combined with a high-fibre carbohydrate food will satisfy the appetite and provide long-term energy, helping to "dilute" the effects that sugar has on your body and to even out unsettling peaks and troughs in blood sugar – ideally negating the desire to snack on sugary foods later on in the day.

Fresh, vibrant and packed with flavour, these healthy main meals have been created to appeal to the whole family, but ingredients can easily be halved to serve a couple of people instead, if desired.

Ribollita

This thick Tuscan soup made with various vegetables and beans is traditionally made a day ahead, hence the name "ribollita", which means "re-boiled" in Italian.

SERVES 4   PREPARATION **15 minutes**   COOKING **35 minutes**

2 tbsp olive oil

1 large onion, roughly chopped

2 leeks, sliced

2 carrots, peeled and sliced

2 celery sticks, sliced

2 large garlic cloves, chopped

2 bay leaves

2 good-sized rosemary sprigs

1.2 litres/44fl oz/5 cups vegetable bouillon

3 large vine-ripened tomatoes, quartered, deseeded and chopped

½ tsp crushed dried chillies

175g/6oz/1½ cups cavolo nero, tough stalks removed and leaves shredded

400g/14oz tin cannellini beans in water, drained and rinsed

salt and freshly ground black pepper

4 heaped tsp black olive tapenade, to serve (optional)

1 Heat the oil in a large saucepan and sauté the onion for 5 minutes, then add the leeks, carrots, celery and garlic and cook for another 4 minutes. Add the bay leaves, rosemary, bouillon, tomatoes and crushed chillies and bring to the boil, then reduce the heat and simmer, half-covered, for 15 minutes.

2 Add the cavolo nero and beans, then cook, half-covered, for a further 10 minutes until the vegetables are tender. Remove a third of the soup and purée in a blender or food processor, then return to the pan.

3 Season the soup to taste and reheat, if necessary, then serve topped with a spoonful of tapenade, if using.

STORAGE
Can be stored in an airtight container in the refrigerator for up to 3 days.

* Health Benefits
Cavolo nero is part of the cabbage family, and, as such, boasts an extraordinary number of health properties. The plant compounds in this group are believed to provide a potent anti-carcinogenic cocktail, stimulating the body's defence system.

Food Facts per Portion
Calories 163kcal • **Total Carbs** 16.5g • **total sugar** 6g • **added sugar** 0g

Lemon & Spinach Lentils with Egg

Puy lentils have a great affinity with mustard, spinach and eggs, and this makes a perfect simple supper dish. Serve with steamed curly kale or cavolo nero.

SERVES 4   PREPARATION **15 minutes**   COOKING **30–35 minutes**

200g/7oz/1 cup Puy or green lentils, rinsed

2 bay leaves

2 tbsp olive oil

2 onions, roughly chopped

4 large/extra-large eggs

4 vine-ripened tomatoes, quartered, deseeded and cut into chunks

225g/8oz/1½ cups spinach, washed, drained well and shredded

3 heaped tsp Dijon mustard

4 tbsp reduced-fat crème fraîche

juice of 1½ lemons

salt and freshly ground black pepper

1   Cover the lentils with cold water in a saucepan, add the bay leaves and bring to the boil, then reduce the heat and simmer, half-covered, for 25–30 minutes until tender but not mushy. Drain the lentils and set aside, discarding the bay leaves.

2   Meanwhile, heat the olive oil in a sauté pan and fry the onions, covered, for 10 minutes until softened. At the same time, bring the eggs gently to the boil in a pan of water and boil for 4 minutes, then remove from the pan. Add the tomatoes and spinach to the onion mixture and cook, stirring, for another 2 minutes until the spinach has wilted.

3   Add the cooked lentils to the pan with the Dijon mustard, crème fraîche and lemon juice, stir until combined and heated through, then season to taste.

4   Spoon the lentils onto 4 plates. Halve the eggs and place on top of the lentils before serving.

STORAGE
The lentil mixture can be stored in an airtight container in the refrigerator for up to 2 days.

* Health Benefits
Like other types of lentil, Puy lentils are a low-fat nutritious source of fibre, protein, folic acid and iron. Eggs are a good source of B vitamins and choline, which have been found to aid brain function.

Food Facts per Portion

Calories 355kcal • **Total Carbs** 28g • **total sugar** 4.45g • **added sugar** 0g

Vegetarian Chilli in Tortilla Baskets

A soft, floury wholemeal tortilla makes a perfect crisp basket when baked, and this can be filled with all manner of goodies – here it is served with a vegetarian chilli.

SERVES 4   PREPARATION **15 minutes**   COOKING **40 minutes**

2 tbsp olive oil, plus extra for brushing

1 large onion, finely chopped

2 tsp cumin seeds

3 large garlic cloves, chopped

1 hot red chilli, halved, deseeded and chopped

1 large red pepper, halved, deseeded and diced

2 courgettes/zucchini, diced

1 tsp ground coriander

½ tsp hot chilli powder

400g/14oz tin kidney beans in water, drained and rinsed

600g/1lb 5oz/2½ cups tinned chopped tomatoes

1 tbsp tomato paste

4 small wholemeal tortillas

4 tsp soured cream

1 small avocado, halved, pitted/stoned, peeled and diced

2 tbsp chopped coriander/cilantro leaves

salt and freshly ground black pepper

1 Heat the oil in a saucepan and sauté the onion for 8 minutes. Stir in the cumin seeds, garlic, chilli, red pepper and courgettes/zucchini and cook for another 5 minutes.

2 Stir in the spices, kidney beans, tomatoes and tomato paste, and bring to the boil, then reduce the heat and simmer, half-covered, for 15 minutes, stirring occasionally. Season.

3 Preheat the oven to 180°C/350°F/Gas 4. Stand 4 heatproof cereal bowls upside down on a baking sheet and brush the base and sides with oil. Carefully drape the tortillas over the top. Bake in the preheated oven for 8–10 minutes until crisp, then remove, leave to cool and lift the tortillas off the bowls.

4 Spoon the chilli into the baked tortilla baskets and top each serving with a spoonful of soured cream, some avocado and a scattering of coriander/cilantro.

STORAGE

The chilli can be stored in an airtight container in the refrigerator for up to 3 days, then reheated.

* Health Benefits

The lycopene in tomatoes protects against heart disease, strokes and destructive free radicals in the nervous system.

Food Facts per Portion

Calories 313kcal • **Total Carbs** 36.4g • **total sugar** 8.6g • **added sugar** 0g

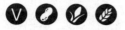

Masoor Dahl

This red lentil dahl can be served as a main dish with lots of green veg and a spoonful of Fresh Coconut Chutney (see page 29).

SERVES 4   PREPARATION **20 minutes**   COOKING **45 minutes**

2 tbsp coconut oil

1 large onion, finely chopped

3 large garlic cloves, chopped

4cm/1½in piece fresh root ginger, peeled and finely chopped

1 tbsp cumin seeds

2 tsp yellow mustard seeds

2 tsp ground coriander

1 tsp hot chilli powder

1 tsp turmeric

10 curry leaves

1 bay leaf

1 large carrot, peeled and diced

140g/5oz/generous ½ cup split red lentils, rinsed

600ml/21fl oz/scant 2½ cups low-salt vegetable bouillon

90ml/3fl oz/heaped ⅓ cup tinned chopped tomatoes

200ml/7fl oz/generous ¾ cup reduced-fat coconut milk

2 tsp fresh lemon juice

1 handful coriander/cilantro leaves, chopped

2 tbsp toasted flaked almonds

salt and freshly ground black pepper

1   Heat half of the oil in a large heavy-based saucepan and fry the onion
    for 10 minutes until softened and beginning to turn golden. Add the
    garlic, ginger, cumin and mustard seeds and cook for 1 minute.

2   Stir in the ground spices, curry leaves, bay leaf, carrot and lentils
    and cook for 1 minute until coated in the spice mixture. Pour in the
    bouillon, chopped tomatoes and coconut milk and bring to the boil,
    then reduce the heat and simmer, half-covered, for 25 minutes, stirring
    occasionally, until the lentils are very tender.

3   Season the lentils to taste and stir in the lemon juice and half of
    the coriander/cilantro. Serve the dahl scattered with the remaining
    coriander and the flaked almonds.

STORAGE
Can be stored in an airtight container in the refrigerator for up to 3 days.

* Health Benefits
*Lentils are small nutritional powerhouses: as well as a useful, low-fat
source of protein, they also provide beneficial amounts of B vitamins,
zinc and iron.*

Food Facts per Portion

Calories 250kcal • **Total Carbs** 26.8g • **total sugar** 7.8g • **added sugar** 0g

Spice-crusted Salmon with Cucumber Salad

The spice crust helps to cut the richness of the salmon and adds plenty of flavour with minimum effort. Serve the salmon with a spoonful of garlicky Tzatziki (see page 31).

SERVES 4　PREPARATION **15 minutes**　COOKING **6–8 minutes**

1 tbsp coriander seeds

1 tbsp cumin seeds

1 tbsp yellow mustard seeds

¼ tsp crushed dried chillies

1 tsp dried thyme

4 salmon fillets, about 150g/5½oz each

1–2 tbsp olive oil

salt and freshly ground black pepper

For the cucumber salad:

1 small cucumber

2 carrots, peeled

1 small red onion, thinly cut into rings

1 tbsp lime juice

2 tsp sesame seeds, toasted

1 Grind the coriander seeds, cumin seeds, mustard seeds and crushed chillies using a pestle and mortar to make a coarse powder, then stir in the thyme and seasoning. Spoon the spice mix over the top of the salmon, pressing it into the fish until you have a thick coating.

2 Heat the oil in a large non-stick frying pan and gently place the fish, spice-crust down, in the pan. Cook for about 6–8 minutes depending on the thickness of the fillet, turning once, until cooked but still pink in the centre.

3 Meanwhile, slice the cucumber and carrots into ribbons using a vegetable peeler. Combine the cucumber, carrots and red onion in a serving dish. Pour over the lime juice, sprinkle with sesame seeds and season to taste.

4 Serve the salmon hot with the salad, or leave until cold.

STORAGE

The cooked salmon can be stored in an airtight container in the refrigerator for up to 2 days.

* Health Benefits

The omega-3 fatty acids found in salmon can help relieve depression, as they appear to enhance the effects of the brain's neurotransmitters that are responsible for mood control.

Food Facts per Portion

Calories 349kcal • **Total Carbs** 2.9g • **total sugar** 2.3g • **added sugar** 0g

Lemon Fish with Salsa Verde

*This simply cooked dish is bursting with fresh summery flavours,
including herbs and lemon. Serve with new potatoes in their skins
and steamed vegetables.*

SERVES 4   PREPARATION **15 minutes**   COOKING **17–20 minutes**

4 thick pollock or haddock fillets, about 175g/6oz each
olive oil, for brushing
8 slices of lemon
salt and freshly ground black pepper

For the salsa verde:
4 tbsp olive oil
2 garlic cloves, minced
1 tbsp capers, drained and rinsed
90ml/3fl oz/heaped ⅓ cup chopped parsley leaves
4 tbsp chopped basil
juice of 1 lemon

1   Preheat the oven to 200°C/400°F/Gas 6. Brush each pollock fillet with
    olive oil. Place each fillet on a piece of foil, large enough to cover the
    fish, and make a parcel.

2   Top each fillet with 2 slices of lemon and season. Fold over the foil to encase the fish, then bake in the preheated oven for 17–20 minutes until just cooked and opaque.

3   Meanwhile, put all the salsa verde ingredients in a blender and process until finely chopped. Season to taste.

4   Remove the parcels from the oven. Carefully unfold each parcel and place the fish on a plate. Drizzle any juices over the top and serve with a spoonful of the salsa verde.

STORAGE

The salsa verde can be stored in an airtight container in the refrigerator for up to 2 days.

* Health Benefits

White fish, such as pollock, have a very low glycaemic index, meaning that they have relatively little impact on blood-sugar levels compared to sugary carbohydrate foods, which cause more severe swings and subsequent uneven energy levels.

Food Facts per Portion

Calories 245kcal • **Total Carbs** 0.8g • **total sugar** 0.5g • **added sugar** 0g

Seafood Hotpot with Rouille

This Spanish-influenced seafood stew is infused with saffron, smoked paprika and garlic. Serve with steamed green vegetables.

SERVES 4   PREPARATION **15 minutes**   COOKING **35 minutes**

2 tbsp olive oil

1 onion, finely sliced

1 red pepper, halved, deseeded and sliced

1 tbsp thyme leaves

2 bay leaves

1 good pinch of saffron

1 tsp smoked paprika

200ml/7fl oz/generous ¾ cup dry white wine

1 courgette/zucchini, sliced

200g/7oz/heaped ½ cup tinned chopped tomatoes

300ml/10½fl oz/1¼ cups low-salt vegetable bouillon

650g/1lb 7oz white fish fillets, skinned and cut into bite-sized pieces

300g/10½oz mixed cooked seafood

salt and freshly ground black pepper

For the rouille:

1 garlic clove, minced

4 tbsp reduced-fat mayonnaise

1 tsp harissa (chilli paste)

1   Combine the rouille ingredients, season to taste and set aside.

2   Heat the oil in a large saucepan and fry the onion for 8 minutes, stirring occasionally. Add the pepper, thyme, bay leaves, saffron and paprika, and cook for 3 minutes. Add the wine and bring to the boil, then cook for about 5 minutes until reduced and the alcohol is burnt off. Reduce the heat, add the courgette/zucchini, tomatoes and bouillon and simmer, half-covered, for 10 minutes.

3   Add the fish and cook for 3 minutes, then add the seafood and heat through for a couple of minutes, stirring gently. Season to taste. Serve in bowls with a spoonful of rouille.

STORAGE

The rouille and sauce can be stored in airtight containers in the refrigerator for up to 2 days. Heat the sauce and continue the recipe from step 3 when ready to serve.

* Health Benefits

Seafood is a good source of zinc, which is a crucial mineral for the brain, immunity, fertility, synthesis of proteins and eyesight.

Food Facts per Portion

Calories 309kcal • **Total Carbs** 5.2g • **total sugar** 4.3g • **added sugar** 0.3g

Thai Mussels with Noodles

Full of fragrant flavours, this curry makes a warming supper dish. Use soba noodles made with buckwheat flour, rather than wheat flour.

SERVES 4   PREPARATION **20 minutes**   COOKING **22 minutes**

200g/7oz dried soba noodles

2 tbsp coconut oil

6 shallots, chopped

3 large garlic cloves, chopped

2 lemongrass stalks, peeled and finely chopped

4 kaffir lime leaves

2 tbsp fish sauce

250ml/9fl oz/1 cup reduced-fat coconut milk

2 heaped tbsp Thai red curry paste, or to taste

2kg/4lb 8oz mussels, scrubbed, cleaned and thoroughly rinsed

juice of 1 lime

1 handful Thai basil leaves

1   Cook the noodles in plenty of boiling water for 3 minutes, then drain and refresh under cold running water and set aside.

2   Heat the oil in a large saucepan and cook the shallots for 5 minutes until softened. Add the garlic, lemongrass and kaffir lime leaves and cook for another minute.

3   Pour in the fish sauce, 200ml/7fl oz/generous ¾ cup water and the
    coconut milk, stir and bring to the boil, then reduce the heat, stir in
    the curry paste and simmer for 5 minutes until reduced.

4   Add the mussels (discarding any that do not shut when tapped), cover,
    and simmer over a medium heat for 5 minutes, shaking the pan
    occasionally, until the mussels have opened. Discard any mussels that
    remain closed. Stir in the lime juice.

5   Divide the noodles between 4 large shallow bowls, spoon the sauce over
    the top, then add the mussels. Sprinkle with basil before serving.

* Health Benefits

*Mussels are an excellent source of minerals, including the antioxidant
selenium, which helps in the production of antibodies and protects the
brain from heavy metals such as mercury used in dental fillings. Mussels
also provide beneficial amounts of vitamin B12, which is vital for the
formation of red blood cells, iron, manganese, phosphorus and zinc – an
important immune booster.*

Food Facts per Portion

Calories 617kcal • **Total Carbs** 51.6g • **total sugar** 5.3g • **added sugar** 0g

Lemon & Prawn Linguine

This light, summery pasta dish is full of fresh flavours and requires little in the way of preparation. You could also try replacing the prawns/shrimp with flakes of cooked salmon. Spelt pasta, which has less gluten but more protein and fibre than regular wheat pasta, is widely available in larger supermarkets and health food stores.

SERVES 4   PREPARATION **10 minutes**   COOKING **15 minutes**

350g/12oz wholegrain spelt linguine

3 courgettes/zucchini, diagonally sliced

200g/7oz/scant 2 cups frozen petits pois

2 tbsp olive oil

2 large garlic cloves, finely chopped

350g/12oz cooked and peeled king prawns/jumbo shrimp

finely grated zest of 1 unwaxed lemon

3 tbsp fresh lemon juice

4 tbsp reduced-fat crème fraîche

1 small handful basil leaves

salt and freshly ground black pepper

1   Cook the pasta in boiling salted water for about 12 minutes until al
    dente. Drain the pasta, reserving 4 tablespoons of the cooking water.

2   Meanwhile, lightly steam the courgettes/zucchini and petits pois until
    just cooked.

3   While the pasta and vegetables are cooking, heat the olive oil in a
    heavy-based saucepan and fry the garlic over a medium-low heat for
    1 minute. Add the prawns/shrimp, lemon zest and juice, crème fraîche
    and reserved water and cook, stirring, for about 1 minute until the
    prawns/shrimp are heated through.

4   Add the pasta, courgettes/zucchini and petits pois, then toss until the
    ingredients are combined and warmed through. Season to taste and
    serve sprinkled with basil leaves.

* Health Benefits
  *Little nuggets of goodness, peas have a high nutritional value when
  compared to their size, providing useful amounts of vitamin C, iron and
  vitamin K. Heart-protecting folic acid and vitamin B6 are also found in
  beneficial amounts.*

Food Facts per Portion
Calories 486kcal • **Total Carbs** 59.9g • **total sugar** 5.7g • **added sugar** 0g

Seared Tuna with Rocket & Tomatoes

This nutritious warm salad provides a perfect combination of protein, carbohydrates and beneficial omega-3 fatty acids. Serve the salad with new potatoes in their skins, if liked.

SERVES 4   PREPARATION **15 minutes**   COOKING **10 minutes**

3 tbsp extra-virgin olive oil

3 tbsp balsamic vinegar

4 thick tuna steaks, about 175g/6oz each

4 vine-ripened tomatoes, halved, deseeded and cut into chunks

200g/7oz tinned chickpeas/garbanzo beans in water, drained and rinsed

2 large handfuls rocket leaves

juice of ½ lemon

salt and freshly ground black pepper

1   Mix together the olive oil and balsamic vinegar and brush a little over the tuna steaks, then season.

2   Heat a griddle pan until very hot. Griddle 2 tuna steaks at a time for about 2 minutes on each side until slightly charred on the outside but still pink in the middle. Cut the tuna into thick slices.

3   Arrange the tomatoes, chickpeas/garbanzo beans and rocket on each plate and top with the tuna. Squeeze over the lemon juice, then drizzle with the remaining olive oil and balsamic dressing. Season to taste, then serve.

STORAGE

The salad and dressing can be stored separately in airtight containers in the refrigerator for up to 1 day. Dress the salad just before serving.

* Health Benefits

Try to include a portion of oily fish, such as tuna, once a week, since the protective effects continue to improve with regular consumption. Fresh tuna is richer in omega-3 fatty acids than tinned.

Food Facts per Portion

Calories 380kcal • **Total Carbs** 9.2g • **total sugar** 3.8g • **added sugar** 0g

Moroccan Chicken Pilaf

You will find ras el hanout, a traditional North African herb and spice mix, in Middle Eastern stores or in some supermarkets. Try cooking the rice in vegetable bouillon to give it extra flavour, and serve the dish with steamed green beans.

SERVES 4   PREPARATION **15 minutes**   COOKING **20 minutes**

2 tbsp olive oil

500g/1lb 2oz skinless, boneless chicken breasts, cut into bite-sized pieces

1 large onion, finely chopped

3 large garlic cloves, chopped

2 tsp cumin seeds

2 bay leaves

5cm/2in piece fresh root ginger, peeled and finely chopped

2 courgettes/zucchini, diced

1 tbsp ras el hanout spice mix

200g/7oz tinned chickpeas/garbanzo beans in water, drained and rinsed

300g/10½oz/scant 2 cups cold cooked brown basmati rice

juice of 1 lime

1 small handful coriander/cilantro leaves, roughly chopped

1 small handful mint leaves, roughly chopped

salt and freshly ground black pepper

1   Heat the oil in a large wok or frying pan. Stir-fry the chicken for
    6 minutes until golden all over, then remove from the wok and
    keep warm.

2   Add the onion and stir-fry for 7 minutes. Next, add the garlic, cumin
    seeds, bay leaves and ginger and stir-fry for another minute. Add the
    courgettes/zucchini, ras el hanout and chickpeas/garbanzo beans, then
    stir-fry for 2 minutes.

3   Add the cooked rice, chicken, lime juice and herbs and stir well as the
    mixture heats through. Season to taste, then serve.

* Health Benefits
*Ras el hanout is typically made up of cardamom, cinnamon, cumin, chilli,
coriander, nutmeg, mace, cloves, peppercorns and turmeric. Spices are
renowned for their digestive and carmitive properties, helping to relieve
indigestion and nausea. Many also have antibacterial qualities.*

Food Facts per Portion
Calories 435kcal • **Total Carbs** 31.8g • **total sugar** 2.3g • **added sugar** 0g

Ginger Chicken Parcels

Cooking foods in a parcel, whether it be foil or baking parchment, helps to retain nutrients and keep moisture in. Here, the chicken is wonderfully succulent and infused with oriental flavours.

SERVES 4   PREPARATION **15 minutes, plus marinating**   COOKING **15–20 minutes**

3 tbsp reduced-salt soy sauce (no added sugar)

1 tbsp toasted sesame oil

1 hot red chilli, halved, deseeded and thinly sliced into rings (optional)

3 tbsp lime juice

625g/1lb 6oz skinless, boneless chicken breasts, cut into 2.5cm/1in-wide strips

5cm/2in piece fresh root ginger, peeled and cut into matchsticks

4 garlic cloves, thinly sliced

6 spring onions/scallions, diagonally sliced

1 large red pepper, halved, deseeded and thinly sliced

1 large carrot, peeled and cut into fine strips

1 tbsp toasted sesame seeds

1   Mix together the soy sauce, sesame oil, chilli, if using, and lime juice in a large shallow dish. Add the chicken and turn until coated in the marinade. Cover the dish and leave to marinate in the refrigerator for at least 1 hour or overnight.

2   Preheat the oven to 200°C/400°F/Gas 6. Using tongs, divide the chicken between 4 pieces of foil, each one large enough to make a parcel. Top the chicken with the ginger, garlic, spring onions/scallions, red pepper and carrot. Spoon the marinade over the top and fold up the foil to make 4 parcels.

3   Place the parcels on a large baking tray and cook in the preheated oven for 15–20 minutes until the chicken is cooked through. Remove from the oven and carefully open the parcels and place on plates. Sprinkle with the sesame seeds before serving.

* Health Benefits
Chicken is rated as a good low-fat source of protein as well as selenium and vitamin B3 (niacin). Research shows that regular consumption of niacin-rich foods such as chicken could provide protection against Alzheimer's disease as well as age-related cognitive decline.

Food Facts per Portion

Calories 299kcal • **Total Carbs** 3.8g • **total sugar** 3.3g • **added sugar** 0g

Chicken with Gazpacho Salsa

Chargrilling is an excellent low-fat method of cooking and gives food a distinctive smoky barbecue flavour. Serve with a watercress salad.

SERVES 4   PREPARATION **15 minutes**   COOKING **25 minutes**

4 skinless, boneless chicken breasts, about 175g/6oz each

olive oil, for brushing

2 tsp paprika

For the gazpacho salsa:

1 yellow pepper, halved, deseeded and cut into small chunks

1 red pepper, halved, deseeded and cut into small chunks

1 small red onion, thinly sliced into rings

1 small cucumber, cut lengthways into quarters, deseeded and cut
  into small chunks

20 pitted/stoned black olives, halved

4 tbsp chopped flat leaf parsley

juice of ½ lemon

1 tbsp extra virgin olive oil

salt and freshly ground black pepper

1   Brush the chicken with olive oil, then sprinkle the paprika evenly
    over each side.

2   Heat a griddle pan until hot. Reduce the heat to medium and griddle the chicken, 2 breasts at a time, for about 6 minutes on each side or until cooked right through. Keep warm while you cook the remaining 2 chicken breasts.

3   Meanwhile, put the yellow and red peppers, red onion, cucumber, olives and parsley in a serving bowl. Pour over the lemon juice and oil, season well and stir until combined.

4   Serve the chicken with the gazpacho salsa by the side.

STORAGE
The gazpacho salsa can be made 1 day in advance and stored in an airtight container in the refrigerator.

* Health Benefits
  Try to eat a range of different coloured vegetables (and fruit) each day to benefit from their range of nutritional attributes. One of the main benefits is that they all contain soluble fibre, which helps to stabilize blood-sugar and blood-cholesterol levels.

Food Facts per Portion
Calories 345kcal • **Total Carbs** 3.6g • **total sugar** 1.3g • **added sugar** 0g

Polpettine in Tomato Sauce

It's extremely quick and easy to make your own meatballs, and the same mixture can be used to make burgers – all without any unwanted additives. You could also swap the turkey mince for chicken, beef or lamb. Serve with wholemeal pasta or rice.

SERVES 4   PREPARATION **20 minutes, plus chilling**   COOKING **20 minutes**

400g/14oz lean turkey mince
55g/2oz/1 cup fresh wholemeal breadcrumbs
1 tsp dried thyme
1 egg, lightly beaten
salt and freshly ground black pepper

For the tomato sauce:
2 tbsp olive oil
3 large garlic cloves, chopped
600g/1lb 5oz/2½ cups tinned chopped tomatoes
1 tbsp tomato paste
2 tsp dried oregano

1   To make the polpettine, mix together the turkey mince, breadcrumbs, thyme, egg and seasoning in a mixing bowl. Form the mixture into 20 walnut-sized balls, then cover and set aside for 30 minutes in the refrigerator to firm up.

2 To make the tomato sauce, heat the oil in a large sauté pan. Fry the garlic for 1 minute, stirring, then add the chopped tomatoes, tomato paste, oregano and seasoning. Bring to the boil, then reduce the heat to a simmer.

3 Carefully add the polpettine to the pan and spoon the sauce over to make sure the balls are covered. Simmer, half-covered, for about 15 minutes until the polpettine are cooked and the sauce reduced, carefully stirring the sauce to prevent it sticking to the bottom of the pan. Serve hot.

STORAGE

The polpettine and tomato sauce can both be stored separately in airtight containers in the refrigerator for 1 day.

* Health Benefits

Turkey, like chicken, is a popular low-fat source of protein, but it is only low-fat without the skin. Along with folic acid, turkey provides a range of B vitamins, a combination that has been found to prevent atherosclerosis.

Food Facts per Portion

Calories 300kcal • **Total Carbs** 15.3g • **total sugar** 5.1g • **added sugar** 0g

Beef & Lentil Curry

This classic rich curry can also be made with lamb. Serve with a wholemeal chapatti and a cucumber and onion salad.

SERVES 4   PREPARATION **15 minutes**   COOKING **65 minutes**

2 tbsp groundnut oil

500g/1lb 2oz lean beef brisket, cut into large bite-sized pieces

2 onions, thinly sliced

3 garlic cloves, chopped

5cm/2in piece fresh root ginger, peeled and grated

4 green cardamom pods, split

2 bay leaves

4 heaped tbsp rogan josh curry paste

200g/3½oz/scant ½ cup tinned chopped tomatoes

6 heaped tbsp tinned green lentils, drained and rinsed

125ml/4fl oz/½ cup natural low-fat bio yogurt

2 tsp fresh lemon juice

1 red chilli, halved, deseeded and sliced (optional)

salt and freshly ground black pepper

1   Heat half of the oil in a large heavy-based saucepan and brown the beef for about 2–3 minutes until the meat is sealed all over, then remove from the pan. You may have to cook the beef in 2 batches. Set the beef aside.

2   If the pan is dry, add the remaining oil (if not, then the extra oil is not needed), then sauté the onions for 8 minutes until softened and golden. Stir in the garlic, ginger, cardamom and bay leaves and cook for 1 minute, then add the curry paste.

3   Pour in 625ml/21fl oz/2½ cups water and the tinned tomatoes, stir and bring to the boil, then reduce the heat, return the beef to the pan and simmer, half-covered, for 45 minutes until the beef is tender.

4   Stir in the lentils, yogurt and lemon juice and cook until heated through. Season to taste, scatter red chilli over the top, if using, then serve.

STORAGE
Can be stored in an airtight container in the refrigerator for up to 3 days.

* Health Benefits

Lean beef can play a part in a healthy diet if eaten in moderation. It is an excellent source of iron, zinc and B vitamins in a readily absorbable form. A lack of iron has been linked with low energy levels, poor concentration, anaemia and learning difficulties.

Food Facts per Portion

Calories 376kcal • **Total Carbs** 19g • **total sugar** 7.4g • **added sugar** 0g

Spiced Beef Kebabs

These kebabs can be grilled/broiled or cooked on the barbecue for a
wonderful smoky flavour. Serve the kebabs and the tahini dip with
a green leaf salad sprinkled with toasted sesame and sunflower seeds.

SERVES 4   PREPARATION **15 minutes, plus marinating**   COOKING **6 minutes**

550g/1lb 4oz lean beef fillet

2 tbsp reduced-salt soy sauce (no added sugar)

1 tbsp sesame oil

1 tbsp olive oil

juice of 1 lime

2.5cm/1in piece fresh root ginger, peeled and grated

1 large garlic clove, minced

½ tsp crushed dried chillies

salt and freshly ground black pepper

For the tahini dip:

125ml/4fl oz/½ cup unsweetened coconut yogurt

2 tbsp light tahini

1 garlic clove, minced

1 medium-hot red chilli, halved, deseeded and finely chopped

1 Flatten the beef with the end of a rolling pin, then cut into 2cm/¾in strips. Mix together the soy sauce, sesame oil, olive oil, lime juice, ginger, garlic and crushed chillies in a large shallow dish. Season well, then add the beef and turn the meat in your hands until it is coated in the marinade. Leave to marinate for at least 1 hour or overnight.

2 While the beef is marinating, make the tahini dip. Mix together the yogurt, tahini, garlic and chilli with 1 tablespoon warm water, then set aside. Preheat the grill/broiler to high.

3 Thread the beef onto 12 skewers (presoaked in water if wooden/bamboo) and cook under the grill for 3 minutes, then turn the kebabs, spoon over the remaining marinade and cook for another 3 minutes.

4 Serve the kebabs with the tahini dip.

* Health Benefits
  Tahini, a paste made from crushed sesame seeds, is a nutritional powerhouse as well as great brain food, being high in vitamins E, B-complex, biotin and choline. It is also rich in protein and calcium, and is reputed to be a better source of these than dairy foods.

Food Facts per Portion
Calories 467kcal • **Total Carbs** 1.4g • **total sugar** 2g • **added sugar** 0g

Ham & Barley Broth

This sustaining and nurturing broth makes a nutritious meal. You could top the broth with grated strong Cheddar, if you like.

SERVES 4   PREPARATION **15 minutes**   COOKING **45 minutes**

100g/3½oz/½ cup pearl barley, rinsed

1 tbsp olive oil

2 onions, sliced

2 celery sticks, sliced

2 large carrots, peeled, halved lengthways and sliced

2 turnips, peeled and cubed

1.2 litres/44fl oz/5 cups low-salt vegetable or chicken bouillon

2 bay leaves

1 bouquet garni

2 rosemary sprigs

150g/5½oz cavolo nero, tough stalks removed and leaves shredded

300g/10½oz thickly cut good-quality ham, diced

salt and freshly ground black pepper

1 Put the pearl barley in a saucepan, cover with water and bring to the boil, then reduce the heat and simmer, covered, for 25 minutes until the pearl barley is soft but not quite cooked.

2 Meanwhile, heat the oil in a large saucepan and sauté the onions, half-covered, for 5 minutes, then add the celery, carrots and turnips. Sauté the vegetables for 5 minutes, then add the bouillon, bay leaves, bouquet garni and rosemary. Bring to the boil, then reduce the heat and simmer for 10 minutes.

3 Drain the pearl barley and add it to the broth with the ham. Simmer, half-covered, for 15 minutes, then add the cavolo nero and cook for a further 5 minutes until it is tender.

4 Season to taste and remove the bay leaves, bouquet garni and rosemary before serving.

Storage
Can be stored in an airtight container in the refrigerator for up to 3 days.

* Health Benefits

Pearl barley is a much underrated grain that provides many nutritional benefits. Alongside cholesterol-lowering fibre, barley provides vitamin B3 (niacin), which has been found to protect against atherosclerosis, the furring up of the arteries.

Food Facts per Portion

Calories 270kcal • **Total Carbs** 34.7g • **total sugar** 5.7g • **added sugar** 0g

Spanish Chorizo & Bean Stew

A great supper for those who don't have much time on their hands and are looking for a meal that is warming and nutritious. Serve with green vegetables and crusty bread for mopping up the sauce.

SERVES 4   PREPARATION 10 minutes   COOKING 25 minutes

1 tbsp olive oil

1 large onion, chopped

250g/9oz chorizo, cut into bite-sized chunks

2 large garlic cloves, chopped

2 tsp dried thyme

400g/14oz/1⅔ cups tinned chopped tomatoes

400g/14oz/1⅔ cups tinned haricot beans in water, drained

2 tsp tomato paste

1 tsp hot smoked paprika

salt and freshly ground black pepper

1   Heat the oil in a large saucepan. Add the onion and fry, stirring, for 7 minutes, then add the chorizo and cook for another 3 minutes. Stir in the garlic and fry for another minute.

2   Add the thyme, tinned tomatoes and beans, tomato paste, paprika and 90ml/3fl oz/generous ⅓ cup water and bring to the boil, stirring occasionally. Reduce the heat and simmer, half-covered, for 10 minutes until the sauce has thickened slightly.

3   Season the stew to taste, then serve in shallow bowls.

STORAGE
Can be stored in an airtight container in the refrigerator for up to 3 days.

* Health Benefits
Although the antiviral, antifungal and antibacterial properties of garlic are most potent when raw, cooking does not inhibit its cancer-protecting, blood-thinning and decongestant properties.

Food Facts per Portion
Calories 314kcal • **Total Carbs** 16.9g • **total sugar** 6.4g • **added sugar** 0g

Marinated Lamb with Chickpea Mash

Chickpeas/garbanzo beans make an excellent alternative to potatoes when mashed, especially when infused with garlic, herbs and the North African spice paste, harissa. Other canned pulses can be used in place of the chickpeas/garbanzo beans when making the mash: try cannellini or haricot beans and prepare them in the same way as the chickpeas/ garbanzo beans. Sumac is a spice that is readily found in Middle Eastern food stores. The spiced lamb is delicious served simply with steamed vegetables such as green beans and broccoli.

SERVES 4   PREPARATION **15 minutes, plus marinating**   COOKING **10–12 minutes**

2 tbsp olive oil

1 tsp paprika

1 tsp dried thyme

1 tsp sumac

4 lean lamb steaks, about 150g/5½oz each

salt and freshly ground black pepper

For the chickpea mash:

2 tbsp olive oil

3 garlic cloves, minced

1 tsp harissa

400g/14oz tin chickpeas/garbanzo beans in water, drained and rinsed

5 tbsp semi-skimmed milk

1 handful coriander/cilantro leaves, chopped

1   Mix together the olive oil, paprika, thyme, sumac and salt and pepper in a large shallow dish. Add the lamb and turn to coat the meat in the marinade, then set aside to marinate for 1 hour.

2   Heat a griddle pan until very hot. Remove the lamb from the marinade and griddle for 6–8 minutes or until cooked to taste, turning halfway through cooking and brushing with the remaining marinade.

3   Meanwhile, to make the chickpea mash, heat the oil in a saucepan and gently fry the garlic for 1 minute, then add the harissa and chickpeas/garbanzo beans and cook for 3 minutes. Stir in the milk to warm through, then transfer everything to a blender or food processor. Purée until smooth and season to taste, then stir in three-quarters of the coriander/cilantro.

4   Divide the chickpea mash between 4 plates and top with the lamb. Scatter with the reserved coriander/cilantro before serving.

* Health Benefits
  The chickpea mash has a lower GI and GL level than mashed potato, meaning that it does not cause such large fluctuations in blood-sugar levels.

Food Facts per Portion
Calories 494kcal • **Total Carbs** 12.4g • **total sugar** 1.4g • **added sugar** 0g

Variation
The spicy marinade can be varied according to personal preference. For a more Mediterranean feel, try a combination of olive oil, 1 tsp dried oregano, 1 tsp dried thyme and ½ tsp smoked paprika. Alternatively, try a combination of olive oil and 1 tsp ground cumin, 1 tsp ground coriander, 1 tsp mild chilli powder and a good squeeze of lemon juice.

DESSERTS

Spiced Chocolate Pots, Mango & Passion Fruit Fool and Baked Vanilla Custards are just a taster of the recipes in this chapter. It doesn't seem possible that these are all low in sugar, but many are low in fat too.

Without putting a damper on things, if following a low-sugar diet you should try to avoid eating dessert every day and see it as an occasional treat, but the good news is that there are numerous naturally sweet foods and alternative flavourings that will help you to create mouthwatering desserts without overloading on sugar or fat.

Importantly, there's no need to resort to artificial sweeteners, with their reported adverse effects on health. Most of the recipes rely on fresh fruit for their natural sweetness as well as natural sweeteners such as brown rice syrup, maple syrup or raw honey. On occasion, xylitol or stevia are used to keep sugar levels as low as feasible.

There is a wide range of desserts to choose from to suit all manner of eating occasion and season, from a summery zingy Melon & Ginger Slush to Popovers with Cherries – perfect comfort food. If time is short, the Superfood Mix, a healthy combination of nuts, berries, raw chocolate and shredded coconut, can almost literally be thrown together in a matter of minutes, and just a handful satisfies a desire for something sweet.

Superfood Mix

On occasion you may not feel like a full-blown dessert, so this combination of nutrient-packed superfoods, including raw chocolate, seeds, nuts and berries, will take the edge off any desire for a little after-dinner sweetness. It also makes a healthy and satisfying snack any time of the day.

SERVES 4   PREPARATION **5 minutes**   COOKING **3–5 minutes**

2 tbsp sunflower seeds
4 tbsp flaked almonds
55g/2oz/scant ½ cup raw cacao nibs
55g/2oz/½ cup goji berries
55g/2oz/scant ½ cup unsweetened desiccated/shredded coconut

1   Toast the sunflower seeds and almonds in a dry frying pan, turning them occasionally, for 3–5 minutes or until starting to turn golden, then leave to cool.

2   Put the sunflower seeds and almonds in a bowl with the cacao nibs,
    goji berries and coconut, then mix until combined.

STORAGE

Can be stored in an airtight container for up to 1 week.

* Health Benefits

*Hailed as the "food of the gods", raw cacao has received considerable
attention recently as it has been found to be one of the richest sources
of antioxidants, exceeding that of red wine and green tea. Raw cacao
does not contain any sugar and is rich in minerals, including sulphur –
which is known as the "beauty mineral" because of its benefits to the skin.
Sulphur has long been recognized for its healing properties, helping to tone
and repair the skin, hair and nails.*

Food Facts per Portion

Calories 295kcal • **Total Carbs** 19.5g • **total sugar** 1.2g • **added sugar** 0g

Variation

Try swapping the almonds for cashew nuts or hazelnuts. Chopped
apricots, raisins or dried cherries make delicious alternatives to the
goji berries.

Fig, Nut & Orange Balls

Packed with energy-giving fruit and nutritious nuts and seeds, these coconut-coated balls make an excellent and different dessert or snack. For a Christmas treat, why not add a splash of brandy to the fruit mixture? Replace 1 tablespoon of the orange juice with the liqueur.

MAKES **about 16**   PREPARATION **20 minutes**   COOKING **5 minutes**

50g/1¾oz/½ cup hazelnuts, roughly chopped

50g/1¾oz/½ cup whole oats

2 tbsp sunflower seeds

2 tbsp pumpkin seeds

70g/2½oz/½ cup raisins

150g/5½oz/scant 1 cup ready-to-eat dried figs, cut into small pieces

4 tbsp fresh orange juice (not from concentrate)

unsweetened desiccated/shredded coconut, for coating

1   Put the hazelnuts and oats in a dry frying pan and toast over a medium heat, turning them frequently, for 5 minutes or until they start to turn golden and the oats become slightly crisp. Leave to cool.

2   Put the nuts, oats and seeds in a food processor or blender and process until finely chopped. Tip the mixture into a mixing bowl.

3   Put the raisins, figs and orange juice into the food processor or blender and purée until the mixture becomes a smooth, thick purée. Scrape the fruit purée into the bowl with the nut mixture and mix until combined. Cover the bowl and chill the mixture for 1 hour.

4   To make the balls, scoop up a portion of the fruit and nut mixture – about the size of a walnut – in a spoon and roll into a ball. Sprinkle the coconut on a plate and roll the ball in it until well coated. Repeat with the remaining mixture to make about 16 balls.

STORAGE

Can be stored in an airtight container for up to 1 week.

* Health Benefits

Dried figs are high in natural sugars so are best not eaten on an everyday basis. They are renowned for their fibre content, helping to relieve constipation and keep the digestive system in good working order. Rich in minerals, figs are also a good source of iron, phosphorus and manganese.

Food Facts per Ball

Calories 88kcal • **Total Carbs** 10.1g • **total sugar** 8.1g • **added sugar** 0g

Fruit & Nut Bars

Packed with protein-rich nuts and seeds as well as energy-giving, iron-boosting dried fruit, one of these simple-to-prepare bars would make a convenient dessert or even breakfast.

MAKES **12 bars**   PREPARATION **15 minutes, plus chilling**   COOKING **3–5 minutes**

25g/1oz/¼ cup hazelnuts, roughly chopped

25g/1oz/¼ cup cashew nuts, roughly chopped

50g/1¾oz/½ cup rolled jumbo oats

2 tbsp sunflower seeds

2 tbsp pumpkin seeds

100g/3½oz/¾ cup raisins

125g/4½oz/scant ¾ cup unsulphured ready-to-eat dried apricots,
   cut into small pieces

4 tbsp fresh orange juice

1   Put the hazelnuts, cashew nuts and oats in a dry frying pan and toast over a medium heat for 3–5 minutes, turning them occasionally with a wooden spatula until they begin to turn golden and the oats become crisp. Remove from the heat and leave to cool.

2   Put the nuts, oats and seeds in a food processor or blender and process until they are very finely chopped. Tip the nut mixture into a bowl.

3   Put the raisins, apricots and orange juice into the food processor or blender and purée until the mixture becomes a smooth, thick purée. Scrape the fruit purée into the mixing bowl and stir into the nut mixture.

4   Line an 18 × 25cm/7 × 10in baking tin/pan with parchment paper. Tip the mixture into the tin and, using a palette knife, smooth into an even layer, about 1cm/½in thick. Chill for 1 hour before cutting into 12 bars.

STORAGE
Can be stored in an airtight container for up to 5 days.

* Health Benefits

Dried fruit is high in natural sugars but, unlike refined sugars, it also provides valuable fibre and nutrients, particularly the mineral iron. The oats, nuts and seeds will all help to slow down the absorption of natural sugars from the dried fruit.

Food Facts per Portion

Calories 110kcal • **Total carbs** 12.8g • **total sugar** 8.9g • **added sugar** 0g

Ⓥ ⓵ Ⓞ ⒅

Apricot & Nut Refrigerator Cake

This "cake" beats store-bought fruit-and-nut chocolate bars hands down. Feel free to use your own favourite fruit and nuts.

MAKES **16 squares**   PREPARATION **15 minutes**   COOKING **12 minutes**

unsalted butter or coconut oil, for greasing
100g/3½oz/generous ½ cup hazelnuts
100g/3½oz/generous ½ cup pecan nuts
55g/2oz/¼ cup blanched whole almonds
150g/5½oz dark/baking chocolate (75% cocoa solids), broken into squares
55g/2oz/scant ½ cup unsweetened dried cherries, roughly chopped
55g/2oz/scant ½ cup unsulphured ready-to-eat dried apricots, chopped
2 egg whites
1 tsp unsweetened cocoa powder, for dusting

1   Lightly grease and line the base of a 20cm/8in square tin/pan. Toast the hazelnuts, pecans and almonds in a large, dry frying pan for 5–6 minutes. (You may have to do this in 2 batches.) Put the hazelnuts in a clean tea towel and rub them to remove their brown papery skins.

2   Melt the chocolate in a heatproof bowl placed over a saucepan of gently simmering water, making sure the bowl does not touch the water. Stir once or twice until melted, then remove from the heat. Leave to cool for 5 minutes, then stir in the nuts, cherries and half of the apricots.

3 Whisk the egg whites in a grease-free mixing bowl until they form
   stiff peaks. Using a metal spoon, stir a spoonful of the whites into the
   chocolate mixture to slacken it, then fold in the remaining egg whites
   until they are well combined.

4 Pour the mixture into the prepared tin, scatter over the remaining
   apricots, then level the top with a palette knife. Refrigerate until solid –
   about 2 hours – then dust with cocoa powder and cut into 16 squares.

STORAGE
Can be stored in an airtight container in the refrigerator for up to 5 days.

* Health Benefits

*There's no getting away from the fact that dried fruit is high in sugar, but
it is not full of empty or nutrient-free calories like refined sugar. In fact,
dried fruit offers many health benefits, namely dietary fibre and a higher
concentration of some vitamins and minerals than its fresh counterpart.
Asthmatics should avoid dried fruit that has been preserved using
sulphites, as it can exacerbate symptoms.*

Food Facts per Portion
Calories 166kcal • **Total Carbs** 10.3g • **total sugar** 9.2g • **added sugar** 5g

Frozen Grapes (plus other fruit)

Fresh fruit take on a whole new existence when frozen and are perfect for a simple dessert that requires very little effort and preparation time. There isn't much to this recipe, but these frozen fruity baubles are really good and convenient. I've allowed 50g/1¾oz per person, but really 1 or 2 grapes is enough to satisfy a desire for a little something sweet. There are also a few variations opposite, which will happily keep in the freezer for several months.

SERVES 4 PREPARATION **5 minutes, plus freezing**

200g/7oz seedless grapes

Put the grapes in a freezer-proof container with a lid or plastic bag and freeze until firm. The grapes can be eaten straight from the freezer or left briefly to soften slightly.

Variations

For easy banana ice cream, peel and wrap a small banana in cling film/ plastic wrap and put in the freezer until frozen. Leave to soften for 10 minutes, then mash with a fork before serving.

For strawberry granita, blend 200g/7oz ripe, hulled strawberries in a blender. Transfer the purée to a freezer-proof container with a lid and freeze until firm. Before serving, transfer the frozen purée to a blender and pulse into ice crystals. Serve straightaway with finely grated lime zest on top.

Storage
Any of these frozen fruit desserts will store in a freezer-proof container or plastic bag in the freezer for up to 3 months.

* Health Benefits
  A reputed detoxifier, grapes are also said to improve the condition of the skin. They are naturally sweet, so are best eaten in moderate amounts.

Food Facts per Portion
Calories 30kcal • **Total Carbs** 6.5g • **total sugar** 6.5g • **added sugar** 0g

Tropical Grapefruit

A refreshing, simple, super-quick dessert that is rich in vitamin C and immune-boosting lycopene. Ginger contains potent antioxidant and anti-inflammatory compounds and adds a warming, aromatic touch to this dish. Select good-quality, organic ground ginger when possible.

SERVES 2   PREPARATION **2 minutes**

1 red grapefruit, halved crossways

1 tsp lime juice

½ tsp ground ginger

2 tsp unsweetened desiccated/shredded coconut (optional)

1   Cut into each grapefruit half with a small, sharp knife to loosen each segment.

2   Spoon the lime juice over each grapefruit half, then sprinkle with the ginger and coconut, if you like. Serve immediately.

* Health Benefits

Grapefruit, especially the pink and red ones, are rich in immune system-boosting antioxidants and also help to reduce harmful LDL cholesterol levels in the body. Eat regularly to reap the benefits of this superfruit.

Food Facts per Portion

Calories 26kcal • **Total Carbs** 5.4g• **total sugar** 5.4g • **added sugar** 0g

Melon & Ginger Slush

This refreshing, zingy granita is just the dessert for a hot summer's day, or it makes a cooling conclusion to a spicy meal.

SERVES 4   PREPARATION **15 minutes, plus freezing**

800g/1lb 12oz ripe honeydew melon, deseeded and skin removed
½ cucumber, peeled, deseeded and chopped
finely shredded zest and juice of 1 lime
4cm/1½in piece fresh root ginger, peeled and grated
2 tsp xylitol or a pinch of stevia, to taste
2 tbsp toasted flaked almonds

1   Put the melon and cucumber in a blender and blend to a coarse purée, then transfer the mixture to a freezer-proof container with a lid. Squeeze the grated ginger through your fingers to extract the juice and stir it into the melon mixture with the lime juice and xylitol. Stir the mixture until combined and taste for sweetness, adding more xylitol if needed.

2   Tip the mixture into a freezer-proof container, cover with the lid and freeze for 2 hours. Remove the container from the freezer and, using a fork, stir to break up the ice crystals. Return to the freezer for another 1½ hours or until frozen.

3   To serve, remove from the freezer and leave to soften for 20 minutes, then scrape the top of the ice with a fork to form loose crystals. Spoon the granita into glasses and top with the flaked almonds and a few strips of lime zest.

STORAGE
Will keep in a freezer-proof container the freezer for up to 3 months.

* Health benefits
  Ginger has long been recognized for its ability to settle the stomach, curbing sickness and nausea, but it has also been found to relieve heartburn, menstrual cramps and cold and flu symptoms.

Food Facts per Portion
Calories 33kcal • **Total Carbs** 4.9 • **total sugar** 4.7g • **added sugar** 0g

Citrus & Pomegranate Salad with Mint

This fruit salad makes a refreshing, invigorating dessert, especially after a spicy meal, as the cooling, calming mint helps to settle the stomach and aids digestion. If you can find red or blood oranges then all the better, since they help to improve glucose tolerance in the body.

SERVES 4   PREPARATION **15 minutes**

1 orange, preferably red or blood

1 red grapefruit

1 ripe pomegranate

1 handful mint leaves, roughly chopped

1   Slice off the skin of the oranges and remove any remaining pith. Thinly slice the oranges into rounds and put them – and any juice – in a serving bowl.

2   Slice off the skin of the grapefruit and remove any pith. Halve the grapefruit crossways and cut into segments. Add to the bowl with any juices.

3   Quarter the pomegranate and remove the arils (seeds). Add to the bowl with any juices. Sprinkle the mint over the fruit just before serving.

STORAGE

Can be covered and stored in the refrigerator for up to 1 day. Add the mint just before serving.

* Health Benefits

Pomegranates are rich in antioxidants, particularly polyphenols, and negate the effect of harmful free radicals. Research shows that the fruit can promote good cardiovascular health and boost the circulatory system. It may reduce the risk of breast cancer as well as lower blood pressure if it is eaten (or the juice drunk) on a daily basis.

Food Facts per Portion

Calories 55kcal • **Total Carbs** 7.6g • **total sugar** 7.4g • **added sugar** 0g

(V) (symbols)

Ricotta with Honey & Walnuts

This must be one of the easiest desserts to make, but its simplicity does not compromise its deliciousness. Protein-rich ricotta is much lower in saturated fat than hard cheese and is a good source of calcium, zinc and mood-enhancing selenium. The drizzle of sweet raw honey and sprinkling of warming cinnamon combine perfectly with the soft, creamy ricotta.

SERVES 4   PREPARATION **5 minutes**   COOKING **4 minutes**

50g/1¾oz/½ cup walnut halves

250g/9oz/1 cup ricotta cheese

100g/3½oz/heaped ½ cup raspberries

2 tsp brown rice syrup, maple syrup or raw honey

½ tsp ground cinnamon

1   Put the walnuts in a large, dry frying pan and toast over a medium heat for about 4 minutes, turning halfway, until they start to colour and smell toasted. Remove from the pan and leave to cool.

2   Place the ricotta on a serving plate. Roughly chop the walnuts and scatter them over the ricotta with the raspberries. Spoon the honey over and sprinkle with the cinnamon. Serve straightaway.

* Health Benefits

Numerous studies highlight the substantial health benefits of walnuts. They are rich in omega-3 fatty acids, which has been found to decrease levels of harmful cholesterol in the body and reduce the risk of heart disease.

Food Facts per Portion

Calories 185kcal • **Total carbs** 6.1g • **total sugar** 4.8g • **added sugar** 2.2g

Mango & Passion Fruit Fool

Fruit fools are a great way of encouraging children to eat more fresh produce, and since the fruit is puréed rather than cooked, it does not lose any of its precious vitamins.

SERVES 4 PREPARATION **10 minutes**

1 ripe mango
300ml/10½fl oz/1¼ cups fromage frais
1 tsp ground allspice
2 passion fruit, halved
8 pecan halves, toasted and roughly chopped

1 Using a vegetable peeler, remove the skin from the mango, then slice the flesh away from the large central stone. Put the mango flesh in a blender and process until puréed.

2 Stir the mango purée and allspice into the fromage frais, then spoon the mixture into 4 glasses.

3   Using a teaspoon, scoop the passion fruit out of its skin, place a
    spoonful on top of each serving and serve sprinkled with the pecans.

STORAGE

Can be covered and stored in the refrigerator for up to 12 hours.

* Health Benefits

*Passion fruit are a good source of immune system-boosting beta carotene
and vitamin C, and the seeds are rich in dietary fibre. The egg-shaped fruit
are also said to have soporific properties.*

Food Facts per Portion

Calories 115kcal • **Total Carbs** 6.9g • **total sugar** 6.9g • **added sugar** 0g

Variation

Berries make great fools and would be a perfect substitute for the mango
and passion fruit. Try a combination of strawberries and raspberries, and
add a scattering of fresh blueberries or blackberries before serving.

Mashed banana or an apple or pear purée also taste delicious stirred
into natural yogurt. Top with some chopped fresh fruit for a variation
in texture.

Prune & Chestnut Fool

Prunes and chestnuts are a classic combination and make the perfect foundation for a deliciously luxurious and creamy fool.

SERVES 4   PREPARATION **10 minutes, plus chilling**   COOKING **6 minutes**

100g/3½oz/½ cup pitted/stoned prunes, chopped

200g/7oz unsweetened chestnut purée

1 tsp vanilla extract

3 tsp brown rice syrup, maple syrup or raw honey

1 tsp xylitol or pinch of stevia, to taste

200ml/7fl oz/generous ¾ cup whipping cream

2 egg whites

1   Put the prunes in a small saucepan with 170ml/5½fl oz/⅔ cup water and bring to the boil, then reduce the heat and simmer, covered, for 5 minutes until very soft. Mash the prunes with the back of a fork in the pan until smooth, then leave to cool.

2   Beat together the chestnut purée, vanilla extract, syrup and xylitol until smooth and combined, then transfer to a mixing bowl. In a separate bowl, whip the cream to soft peaks. Fold the cream into the chestnut mixture until combined.

3   Whisk the egg whites in a grease-free bowl until they form stiff peaks. Using a metal spoon, stir a spoonful of the whites into the chestnut mixture to slacken it, then fold in the remaining egg whites until they are well combined.

4   Gently stir in the prune purée to give a swirled effect, then spoon into 4 glasses and serve.

STORAGE

Can be stored in the refrigerator for up to 2 days.

* Health Benefits

Prunes are well known for their ability to prevent constipation thanks to their high fibre content. Chestnuts contain less fat than other nuts, and it is mostly the unsaturated type. They are also the only nut that provides vitamin C.

Food Facts per Portion

Calories 232kcal • **Total Carbs** 14g • **total sugar** 9g • **added sugar** 3.3g

Spiced Chocolate Pots

*Chocolate and spices are perfect partners. This chocolate mousse tastes
very indulgent and makes a special dinner party dessert. If you can't find
the natural sweetener lucuma powder in health food stores or online, you
can swap it for brown rice syrup, maple syrup or raw honey.*

SERVES 4   PREPARATION **15 minutes, plus chilling**   COOKING **5 minutes**

50g/1¾oz dark/baking chocolate (75% cocoa solids), broken into squares

2 eggs, separated

1 tbsp xylitol or large pinch of stevia, to taste

2 tsp lucuma powder

1 tsp ground allspice

¾ tsp ground cinnamon

1 tsp vanilla extract

4 tbsp double/heavy cream

1   Melt the chocolate in a heatproof bowl placed over a saucepan of gently
     simmering water, making sure the bottom of the bowl does not touch
     the water. Leave to cool for 5 minutes.

2   Meanwhile, whisk the egg whites in a grease-free bowl until they
    form soft peaks. Add the xylitol and continue to whisk to form stiff,
    glossy peaks.

3   Beat the egg yolks, lucuma, allspice, cinnamon, vanilla and cream
    into the chocolate mixture. Using a metal spoon, stir a spoonful of
    the whites into the chocolate mixture to slacken it, then fold in the
    remaining egg whites until they are well combined.

4   Spoon the chocolate mousse into 4 ramekins or small glasses, then
    chill for 30 minutes until set.

STORAGE

Can be covered and stored in the refrigerator for up to 2 days.

* Health Benefits

*If eaten in moderation, chocolate is good for us, and the darker and higher
in cocoa solids the better. Rich in flavonoids, which act as antioxidants,
a small amount of dark/baking chocolate eaten every day can benefit
the heart, reduce blood pressure and lower LDL cholesterol levels. It also
stimulates endorphin production, making you feel good.*

Food Facts per Portion

Calories 266kcal • **Total Carbs** 11.7g • **total sugar** 4g • **added sugar** 1.3g

Horchata

This version of the popular Spanish almond drink comes with a twist. Along with the usual cinnamon stick to flavour the milk, the recipe includes cloves, nutmeg and star anise, which add a slight sweetness. It can be served chilled or warm as a simple dessert or comforting bedtime drink and is just the thing to satisfy a craving for something sweet.

SERVES 2   PREPARATION **10 minutes**   COOKING **5 minutes**

½ recipe quantity (about 500ml/17fl oz/2 cups) Almond Milk (see page 34)

1 cinnamon stick

4 cloves

1 star anise

½ tsp freshly grated nutmeg, plus extra to serve

1 tsp vanilla extract

1 tsp brown rice syrup, maple syrup or raw honey

ice, to serve (optional)

1   Put the almond milk in a small pan and add the cinnamon, cloves, star anise and nutmeg. Heat gently until the milk almost comes to the boil, then leave to infuse for 30 minutes.

2   Pick out the spices and stir in the xylitol, to taste. The horchata can be reheated until warm or served cold or chilled with ice. A sprinkling of extra nutmeg adds the finishing touch.

STORAGE

Can be stored in an airtight container in the refrigerator for up to 2 days.

* Health Benefits

Studies show that cinnamon may have a regulatory effect on blood-sugar levels, making it particularly useful for those with Type 2 diabetes. Its natural sweet flavour helps to curb sugar cravings, too.

Food Facts per Portion

Calories 157kcal • **Total Carbs** 5.5g • **total sugar** 4.7g • **added sugar** 2.2g

Banana Griddle Cakes

Banana helps to add a touch of sweetness to these griddle cakes,
replacing the need for refined sugar. Serve sprinkled with fresh berries
and a spoonful of fromage frais.

SERVES 4   PREPARATION **25 minutes**   COOKING **10–14 minutes**

140g/5oz/1¼ cups self-raising wholemeal flour
1 tsp baking soda
200ml/7fl oz/generous ¾ cup almond milk
1 egg, lightly beaten
2 heaped tbsp natural low-fat bio yogurt
1 large, ripe banana, mashed
coconut oil, for frying

1   Sift the flour (adding any bran left in the sieve) and baking soda into a
    mixing bowl and make a well in the centre.

2   Whisk the milk with the egg, then gradually pour it into flour,
    whisking constantly to avoid any lumps. Stir in the yogurt and set aside
    for 15 minutes, then stir in the mashed banana.

3   Heat a flat griddle or large non-stick frying pan, then dip a scrunched-up piece of kitchen paper into the oil and carefully wipe a little over the pan. Spoon 3 tablespoons of the batter per cake into the pan, cooking 3 cakes at a time, and cook for about 1–1½ minutes on each side until golden. Remove and keep warm, then re-oil the pan before cooking the remaining 3 batches of cakes to make a total of 12. Serve the griddle cakes warm.

STORAGE

The griddle cakes can be stored in an airtight container in the refrigerator for up to 1 day, then reheated.

* Health Benefits

  The fibre found in wholemeal flour and bananas helps to slow the digestion and absorption of carbohydrates, including sugars, in the body, which means that blood-glucose levels remain stable after eating.

Food Facts per Portion

Calories 200kcal • **Total Carbs** 12.3g • **total sugar** 7.4g • **added sugar** 0g

Chocolate & Cardamom Pudding

*This nutritious alternative to rice pudding is made with protein-rich
quinoa flakes and flavoured with raw cacao, cardamom and cinnamon.
It can be served warm or left to cool.*

SERVES 4   PREPARATION **5 minutes**   COOKING **15 minutes**

900ml/32fl oz/3¼ cups unsweetened almond milk

120g/4¼oz/generous ½ cup quinoa flakes

3–4 green cardamom pods, to taste, split

1 heaped tsp ground cinnamon

1 tsp freshly ground nutmeg, plus extra to serve

3 tbsp raw cacao powder

2 tsp vanilla extract

2 tsp xylitol or pinch of stevia, to taste

2 tsp brown rice syrup, maple syrup or raw honey

1 tbsp toasted flaked almonds, for sprinkling

1   Put the almond milk in a medium-sized pan and stir in the quinoa
    flakes, cardamom, cinnamon, nutmeg, raw cacao powder, vanilla extract
    and xylitol until combined.

2   Bring the milk up to simmering point, then cook, stirring regularly,
    for 12–15 minutes until thickened. Stir in the syrup and divide into
    4 serving bowls. Grate a little extra nutmeg over the top and serve
    sprinkled with the almonds.

STORAGE

Can be stored covered in the refrigerator for up to 3 days.

* Health Benefits
*Almonds are rich in vitamin E. This antioxidant decreases the risk of
cataracts and coronary heart disease. The heart also benefits from the
nut's monounsaturated fat content, which has been found to reduce levels
of LDL cholesterol.*

Food Facts per Portion

Calories 283kcal • **Total Carbs** 26.5g • **total sugar** 2.8g • **added sugar** 2.2g

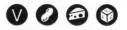

Baked Figs with Vanilla Cream & Almonds

Fresh figs are bursting with nutrients and are delicious baked in a rich, orangey syrup. Accompanying them with a good dollop of vanilla cream and a sprinkling of toasted almonds creates a delicious dessert.

SERVES 4   PREPARATION **15 minutes**   COOKING **15 minutes**

4 fresh, not too ripe, figs

finely grated zest and juice of 1 orange

few drops orange flower water (optional)

1 tbsp brown rice syrup, maple syrup or raw honey

2 heaped tbsp flaked almonds

125ml/4fl oz/½ cup 2% fat Greek yogurt

1 tsp vanilla extract

1   Preheat the oven to 180°C/350°F/Gas 4. Stand the figs upright and cut each one into quarters, but do not cut right through to the base. Place the figs in an ovenproof dish, making sure they stand upright.

2   Mix together the orange juice, orange flower water, if using, and the syrup and spoon it over the figs. Scatter the orange zest over the top. Bake in the preheated oven for 15 minutes until softened.

3   Meanwhile, put the flaked almonds in a dry frying pan and toast them for about 3 minutes or until light golden.

4   Mix together the yogurt and vanilla in a bowl until combined.

5   Remove the figs from the oven and divide between 4 bowls, then spoon any juices over the top. Sprinkle with the toasted almonds and add a spoonful of the vanilla cream, then serve.

STORAGE

The vanilla cream can be stored in an airtight container in the refrigerator for up to 2 days.

* Health Benefits

Figs are a well-known laxative, which is due to their high fibre content. Fibre also plays a beneficial part in protecting the heart and in weight control. The fruit is also rich in potassium, a mineral that helps to control blood pressure, and calcium, which is vital for protecting bone density. In fact, these minerals work in tandem to protect and strengthen the bones and teeth.

Food Facts per Portion

Calories 198kcal • **Total Carbs** 11.8g • **total sugar** 7.5g • **added sugar** 3g

Plum Brûlées

This version of the classic crème brûlée makes the perfect dessert for a special occasion. It is topped with a fine sprinkling of unrefined coconut sugar, to give the classic caramelized top. This low GI sweetener is a good source of minerals and B vitamins and makes a suitable alternative to regular brown cane sugar. Spray a mist of water over the brûlées before grilling/broiling to encourage the caramelization of the sugar.

SERVES 4   PREPARATION **15 minutes**   COOKING **10–12 minutes**

6 ripe dark red plums, such as mirabelle, pitted/stoned and chopped
125ml/4fl oz/½ cup 2% fat Greek yogurt
125ml/4fl oz/½ cup unsweetened coconut yogurt
½ tsp vanilla extract
2 tsp coconut palm sugar

1   Put the plums in a saucepan with 2 tablespoons water and bring to the boil, then reduce the heat and simmer, half-covered, for 5 minutes until softened.

2   Mash the plums with the back of a fork in the pan until the fruit is mushy. Divide the plums into 4 ramekins, then leave the fruit to cool.

3 Preheat the grill/broiler to high. Mix together the Greek yogurt, coconut yogurt and vanilla extract, then spoon the mixture on top of the plums, dividing it equally between each ramekin. Sprinkle ½ teaspoon coconut sugar over the top of each serving.

4 Place the brûlées in a grill/broiler pan and cook under the preheated grill/broiler for 3–5 minutes until golden and caramelized – keeping an eye on them as the sugar can burn easily. Leave to cool for 5 minutes or completely before serving.

STORAGE
Can be covered and stored in the refrigerator for up to 1 day. Alternatively, cover the brûlées before sprinkling and grilling/broiling them, and store for up to 2 days in the refrigerator.

* Health Benefits
Vitamin C is found in useful amounts in plums, which, along with assisting in the absorption of iron, is needed by the body to make healthy tissue, support the immune system and protect against damage caused by harmful free radicals.

Food Facts per Portion
Calories 106kcal • **Total Carbs** 10.8g • **total sugar** 8.6g • **added sugar** 2.2g

Ⓥ 🥜 🌙 🔺 🎲

Raspberry Yogurt Creams

Yummy creamy, custardy fruit pots: this simple and easy-to-prepare dessert ticks all the right boxes if you are looking for something sweet – but not too sweet! The sharpness of the raspberries cuts through the creaminess and the fruit provides a good hit of vitamin C, plus plenty of antioxidant and anti-inflammatory phytonutrients.

SERVES 4   PREPARATION **10 minutes**   COOKING **12–14 minutes**

2 tbsp flaked almonds

2 tbsp sunflower seeds

2 egg yolks

250ml/9fl oz/1 cup unsweetened coconut yogurt

1½ tsp vanilla extract

tsp brown rice syrup, maple syrup or raw honey

1 tsp xylitol or pinch of stevia, to taste

150g/5½oz/scant 1 cup raspberries

1   Lightly toast the almonds and sunflower seeds in a dry frying pan until light golden, taking care not to let them burn, then set aside.

2   Put the egg yolks, yogurt, vanilla extract, syrup and xylitol in a medium, heavy-based saucepan and heat gently, stirring frequently, until the mixture starts to bubble. Reduce the heat slightly and continue to stir for about 10–12 minutes until the mixture thickens to the consistency of custard.

3   Divide the raspberries into 4 ramekins. Spoon the custard over the top and serve sprinkled with the almonds and sunflower seeds.

STORAGE

The raspberries and custard can be covered and stored in the refrigerator for 2 days. Add the nuts and seeds just before serving.

* Health Benefits

The humble almond has numerous health attributes: it is rich in monounsaturated fats, vitamin E and antioxidants. These combine to reduce harmful LDL cholesterol in the body and raise beneficial HDL cholesterol, which helps to reduce the risk of heart disease and strokes.

Food Facts per Portion

Calories 210kcal • **Total Carbs** 9.5g • **total sugar** 5.7g • **added sugar** 2.1g

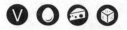

Baked Vanilla Custards

Spices are a great way of adding flavour and a natural sweetness to desserts, negating the need for lots of sugar. For the best flavour, choose pure vanilla extract rather than vanilla flavouring.

SERVES 4   PREPARATION **15 minutes**   COOKING **45 minutes**

300ml/10½fl oz/scant ½ cup milk

1 star anise

1 tsp ground cinnamon

2 eggs

1 tbsp xylitol or pinch of stevia, to taste

1 tbsp brown rice syrup, maple syrup or raw honey

1 tsp vanilla extract

freshly grated nutmeg, for sprinkling

1   Preheat the oven to 170°C/325°F/Gas 3. Put the milk, star anise and cinnamon in a small pan and heat almost to boiling point, stirring occasionally. Remove from the heat and leave for 10 minutes to infuse the milk with the spices.

2   Meanwhile, whisk together the eggs and xylitol until pale and creamy. When the milk has had time to infuse, reheat it to almost boiling point. Strain the milk into the egg mixture, then add the vanilla extract and stir well until combined. Discard the star anise.

3   Pour the custard into 4 large ramekins and put them in a baking tin/ pan. Pour enough just-boiled water to come two-thirds of the way up the sides of the ramekins. Carefully put the tin/pan in the oven and bake for 30–35 minutes, or until the custards have set but are still a little wobbly. Grate over a little nutmeg and serve warm or leave until cold.

STORAGE

Can be covered and stored in the refrigerator for up to 2 days.

* Health Benefits

Studies have shown that just ½ teaspoon cinnamon a day can help to reduce harmful LDL cholesterol in the body. There is also evidence to suggest that cinnamon can moderate blood-sugar levels, making it especially beneficial for those with Type 2 diabetes.

Food Facts per Portion

Calories 110kcal • **Total Carbs** 9.5g • **total sugar** 6.5g • **added sugar** 3.3g

Sweet Soufflé Omelette

It may not be an obvious dessert, but an omelette tastes just as delicious with a sweet filling as a savoury one. You could try stewed plums or berries instead of the apple filling.

SERVES 2   PREPARATION **15 minutes**   COOKING **15 minutes**

1 large sweet apple, peeled, cored and diced
½ tsp ground cinnamon
2 large/extra-large eggs, separated
1 tsp xylitol or pinch of stevia, to taste
5g/¼oz/1 tsp unsalted butter or coconut oil

1   Put the apple in a medium saucepan with 4 tablespoons water and
    the cinnamon. Bring to the boil, then reduce the heat and simmer,
    covered, for 8 minutes or until tender. Mash lightly with a fork to make
    a chunky purée, then set aside.

2   Whisk the egg whites in a grease-free bowl until they form stiff peaks.
    Whisk the egg yolks separately until they are even in colour and
    texture, then stir in the xylitol. Carefully fold the egg whites into the
    egg yolks using a metal spoon.

3   Melt the butter in a large non-stick frying pan and swirl it around
    to cover the base. Tip the frothy egg mixture into the pan and gently
    flatten with a spatula (without losing too much air) until it covers
    the base of the pan. Cook over a medium heat for 2–3 minutes until
    light golden.

4   Spoon the apple down the centre of the omelette, cook for another
    minute, then fold it in half to encase the fruit. Slide the omelette on
    to a serving plate, cut in half crossways and serve.

STORAGE

The apple purée can be stored in an airtight container in the refrigerator for up
to 3 days.

* Health Benefits

*Cinnamon lends a pleasing warmth to sweet and savoury dishes. It has
antibacterial properties and has been found to reduce both blood-glucose
and unhealthy fat levels if eaten on a regular basis.*

Food Facts per Portion

Calories 127kcal • **Total Carbs** 11.1g • **total sugar** 8g • **added sugar** 0g

Ricotta Cakes with Berry Sauce

These orange-infused ricotta puddings come with a simple berry sauce.
Make sure you buy good-quality ricotta for the best texture and flavour.

SERVES 4   PREPARATION **15 minutes**   COOKING **20 minutes**

olive oil, for greasing

280g/10oz/1¼ cups ricotta cheese

1 tbsp xylitol or pinch of stevia, to taste

finely grated zest of 1 orange

2 large/extra-large egg whites

300g/10½oz/2½ cups mixed fresh or frozen berries, defrosted if frozen

4 tbsp fresh orange juice (not from concentrate)

1 star anise

1   Preheat the oven to 180°C/350°F/Gas 4. Lightly grease 4 dariole moulds.
    Using a wooden spoon, beat together the ricotta, xylitol and orange zest
    in a mixing bowl.

2   Whisk the egg whites in a grease-free bowl until they form soft
    peaks. Using a metal spoon, stir a spoonful of the whites into the
    ricotta mixture to slacken it, then fold in the remaining egg whites
    until they are well combined. Spoon the mixture into the moulds.
    Bake in the preheated oven for about 20 minutes or until risen and
    light golden.

3   Meanwhile, to make the berry sauce, put three-quarters of the fruit in a saucepan with the orange juice and star anise, then heat gently for 3–5 minutes until the berries are soft and juicy. Press the fruit through a sieve to remove the pips and star anise.

4   Remove the moulds from the oven and leave to cool slightly, then carefully turn out the ricotta cakes and place them on plates. Serve warm with the sauce and decorate with the reserved berries.

STORAGE

The cakes can be stored in an airtight container in the refrigerator for up to 2 days and the fruit sauce for up to 5 days.

* Health Benefits

Make use of spices, such as star anise, cinnamon and nutmeg, to add flavour and aroma to sweet and savoury dishes. As well as their antibacterial and digestive benefits, they reduce the need for large quantities of added sugar.

Food Facts per Portion

Calories 154kcal • **Total Carbs** 11.8g • **total sugar** 6.6g • **added sugar** 0g

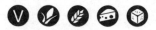

Strawberry Filo Tarts

These pretty little tarts are filled with strawberries and a luxurious – and low-fat – creamy filling. What's more, they look impressive but are surprisingly easy to make for a special dinner party dessert.

SERVES 4   PREPARATION **20 minutes**   COOKING **20 minutes**

25g/1oz/4½ tsp unsalted butter or coconut oil, melted
4 filo pastry sheets, each about 30 × 18cm/12 × 7in

For the filling:
8 heaped tbsp quark
1 tsp vanilla extract
4 tsp brown rice syrup, maple syrup or raw honey
12 strawberries, halved if large

1   Preheat the oven to 180°C/350°F/Gas 4. Using a little of the melted butter or oil, lightly grease 4 holes in a deep muffin tin/pan. Cut each sheet of filo into three 10cm/4in squares, so you have 12 squares in total. Discard any surplus pastry.

2   Carefully press a square of filo into each hole in the muffin tin/pan and lightly brush with melted butter, then layer 2 more sheets on top, brushing with more butter as you go. Layer each one diagonally so that you end up with baskets each with a 12-point star top.

3   Bake the baskets in the preheated oven for about 20 minutes until golden and crisp, then remove from the oven and leave to cool.

4   To make the filling, beat together the quark, vanilla extract and syrup. Spoon the creamy mixture into the filo cups and top with the strawberries. Serve immediately.

STORAGE

The baked unfilled filo baskets can be stored in an airtight container in the refrigerator for up to 3 days and the cream filling for up to 2 days.

* Health Benefits

Strawberries contain a unique combination of antioxidant phenols, including ellagic acid and anthocyanins, to protect us from heart disease, certain cancers and age-related macular degeneration. Strawberries also contain plentiful amounts of fibre, vitamin C, manganese and potassium and have anti-inflammatory and glucose-balancing properties.

Food Facts per Portion

Calories 111kcal • **Total Carbs** 10g • **total sugar** 6.5g • **added sugar** 4.5g

Variation

Use blueberries or raspberries instead of the strawberries, and you can also top the tarts with unsweetened desiccated/shredded coconut.

Stuffed Pistachio Peaches

In this deliciously moreish, quick pudding, the peaches are stuffed with
a creamy, nutritious date and nut filling. Nectarines can be used as an
alternative to peaches.

SERVES 4   PREPARATION **10 minutes**   COOKING **6–7 minutes**

4 tbsp low-fat cream cheese

2 tbsp fresh orange juice (not from concentrate)

finely grated zest of ½ orange

½ tsp vanilla extract

2 ripe peaches, halved and pitted/stoned

40g/1½oz/scant ½ cup unsalted pistachio nuts or other favourite nuts,
    roughly chopped

freshly grated nutmeg, for sprinkling

1   Preheat the grill/broiler to medium and line the grill pan with foil. Mix together the cream cheese, orange juice, orange zest and vanilla in a small bowl.

2   Spoon the cream cheese mixture into the hollows in the peach halves, then cook for 6–7 minutes under the preheated grill/broiler until the filling starts to turn golden and the fruit softens.

3   Remove from the grill/broiler, scatter the pistachio nuts on top and sprinkle with a little nutmeg. Serve straightaway. Alternatively, serve at room temperature, but add the pistachios and nutmeg only when ready to serve.

* Health Benefits

Much of the vitamin C content of a peach is found just below the skin, so the fruit is most nutritious when served unpeeled. Peaches are also a good source of the antioxidant beta carotene, which is converted to vitamin A in the body.

Food Facts per Portion

Calories 160kcal • **Total Carbs** 6.8g • **total sugar** 6.1g • **added sugar** 0g

(V) (O) (✿) (✿) (▦) (⬦)

Popovers with Cherries

This idea of serving Yorkshire puddings as a dessert is a novel one,
but with the cherry topping this is similar to a low-sugar version of
the French clafoutis. Serve with a spoonful of low-fat crème fraîche.

SERVES 6   PREPARATION **10 minutes, plus resting**   COOKING **20 minutes**

115g/4oz/1 cup plain/all-purpose flour
½ tsp baking powder
pinch of salt
70ml/2¼fl oz/scant ⅓ cup semi-skimmed milk
1 egg, lightly beaten
2 tsp sunflower oil

For the filling:
200g/7oz/heaped 1 cup dark cherries, pitted/stoned
3 tsp brown rice syrup, maple syrup or raw honey
freshly grated nutmeg, to decorate

1   Sift the flour, baking powder and salt into a mixing bowl and make a
    well in the centre. Put 4 tablespoons water and the milk in a jug, add
    the egg and whisk until combined. Pour the egg mixture into the bowl,
    then gradually whisk together to make a thin batter. Pour the mixture
    into the jug and set aside for 20 minutes.

2   Preheat the oven to 220°C/425°F/Gas 7. Pour a little oil into each cup of a 6-hole deep muffin tin/pan, then put the tin/pan in the preheated oven for 8 minutes until very hot. Carefully remove from the oven and pour the batter into the holes. Return to the oven for 20 minutes until risen and golden.

3   Meanwhile, put the cherries in a saucepan with 100ml/3½fl oz/scant ½ cup water, cover and cook over a medium-low heat for 5 minutes until softened.

4   Remove the popovers from the oven and serve 1 per person, topped with the cherries. Drizzle with the syrup and grate over a little nutmeg. Serve straightaway.

* Health Benefits
With their ability to cleanse the body by removing toxins from the kidneys, cherries are said to benefit those who suffer from gout and arthritis. Cherries also contain iron, potassium and vitamins C and B.

Food Facts per Portion
Calories 105kcal • **Total Carbs** 19g • **total sugar** 6.4g • **added sugar** 1.7g

CAKES, BAKES & BREADS

This deliciously diverse collection of recipes shows that it is possible to make delicious cakes, cookies and baked treats with the minimum amount of added sugar. This doesn't mean that they should form an everyday part of your diet though; the saying "everything in moderation" is key here! The occasional slice of Spiced Apple Cake, helping of Apple & Raspberry Flapjack Pie or square of Chocolate & Beetroot Brownie make a welcome treat and will satisfy any desire for something sweet without you having to overindulge. You'll find low-sugar versions of family favourites, such as muffins, cheesecake, cookies and shortbread; what's more, many are surprisingly lower in fat than their regular counterparts.

When baking, fruit will help to keep your cakes moist as well as add natural sweetness and substance, while spices such as nutmeg and cinnamon add a wonderful aroma and flavour. Unlike refined sugar and its empty calories, fruit provides valuable fibre as well as a range of vitamins and minerals. Where necessary, but not to excess, xylitol, stevia and brown rice syrup are also used. These natural sugar alternatives do not cause irregular blood-sugar levels in the same way as refined sugar does, while the fibre in fruit also helps to curb peaks and troughs.

The chapter also includes a few savoury recipes, as well as the simplest bread in the world to make – soda bread made with the wonderfully nutty-flavoured wholemeal spelt flour. Enjoy!

Coconut, Banana & Oat Cookies

Free from added sugar, these cookies get their sweetness from the bananas, coconut and raw cacao nibs.

MAKES 20   PREPARATION **15 minutes**   COOKING **15–20 minutes**

butter or coconut oil, for greasing

100g/3½oz/1 cup rolled jumbo oats

50g/1¾oz/scant ⅓ cup ground almonds

100g/3½oz/1 cup unsweetened desiccated/shredded coconut

¼ tsp ground cinnamon

½ tsp baking powder

2 large ripe bananas, peeled

½ tsp vanilla extract

5 tbsp coconut oil or olive oil, warmed until liquid

100g/3½oz/generous ½ cup raw cacao nibs

1   Preheat the oven to 180°C/350°F/Gas 4. Lightly grease 2 large baking sheets.

2   In a large mixing bowl, mix together the oats, ground almonds, coconut, cinnamon and baking powder.

3   In a second bowl, mash the bananas well, then stir in the vanilla
    extract and warmed coconut oil. Add the wet ingredients to the dry
    ingredients and mix well, then fold in the raw cacao nibs.

4   Place 20 tablespoons of the dough onto the prepared baking sheets, and
    flatten the tops slightly to make cookies about 4cm/1½in in diameter.

5   Bake in the preheated oven for 15–20 minutes until golden. Remove
    from the oven and leave to cool for a few minutes, then transfer to a
    wire rack to cool.

STORAGE

Can be stored in an airtight container for up to 5 days.

* Health Benefits

*The numerous health properties of coconut oil can be attributed to the
presence of lauric, capric and caprylic acids, which are antimicrobial,
antioxidant, antifungal and antibacterial. There is a whole string of
associated benefits, including reduced risk of kidney problems, heart
disease, high blood pressure, diabetes and cancer. There are also recorded
improvements in the condition of the hair, skin, bone strength, metabolism
and digestion. Use organic virgin oil rather than a blended variety.*

Food Facts per Cookie

Calories 124kcal • **Total Carbs** 7.9g• **total sugar** 2.5g • **added sugar** 0g

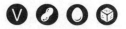

Coconut Macaroons

So simple and yet so good... these coconut cookies are incredibly quick and easy to rustle up and are perfect with an afternoon cup of tea or coffee. They also make great party food, for both adults and children, as unlike regular store-bought macaroons, they aren't laden with added sugar and other additives. If using coconut oil, make sure you opt for organic virgin oil.

MAKES 15   PREPARATION 10 **minutes**   COOKING 12 **minutes**

unsalted butter or coconut oil, for greasing
3 egg whites
40g/1½oz/scant ¼ cup xylitol
110g/3¾oz/generous 1¼ cups unsweetened desiccated/shredded coconut

1   Preheat the oven to 180°C/350°F/Gas 4 and lightly grease 2 non-stick
      baking trays/tins or line with parchment paper.

2   Lightly whisk the egg whites in a large, grease-free mixing bowl until frothy and bubbly, then fold in the xylitol and coconut until combined.

3   Place 15 tablespoons of the coconut mixture on the baking trays/ tins and flatten the tops slightly with the back of a spoon. Bake for 10–12 minutes until just beginning to turn golden.

4   Leave to cool slightly before transferring them to a wire rack to cool.

STORAGE

Can be stored in an airtight container for up to 3 days.

* Health Benefits

Coconuts are rich in lauric acid, which is known to for its antibacterial, antiviral and antifungal properties. Coconuts are also said to raise levels of beneficial HDL cholesterol in the body.

Food Facts per Macaroon

Calories 26kcal • **Total Carbs** 3.6g • **total sugar** 0.4g • **added sugar** 0g

Ⓥ ⬤ ⬤ ⬤ ⬤

Almond & Raw Chocolate Drops

These moist, coconutty cookies have a slight crunch thanks to the raw cacao nibs. Keep an eye on them when they're baking as they can brown too quickly; you want them a light golden colour.

MAKES 12   PREPARATION **10 minutes**   COOKING **12 minutes**

100g/3½oz/scant 1 cup ground almonds
20g/¾oz/scant ¼ cup raw cacao nibs
30g/1oz/¼ cup unsweetened desiccated/shredded coconut
½ tsp baking powder
pinch of salt
30g/1oz/scant ¼ cup xylitol
1 tbsp brown rice syrup, maple syrup or raw honey
1 egg, separated
3 tbsp coconut oil, melted
½ tsp vanilla extract

1   Preheat the oven to 180°C/350°F/Gas 4. Line a baking sheet with parchment paper.

2   Mix together the ground almonds, cacao nibs, coconut, baking powder, salt and xylitol in a mixing bowl.

3   Add the syrup, egg yolk, coconut oil and vanilla extract and mix until well combined.

4   Whisk the egg white in a grease-free mixing bowl until it forms soft peaks, then fold it into the almond mixture to make a soft dough.

5   Place 12 walnut-sized balls of the dough onto the prepared baking sheet, and flatten the tops slightly to make cookies about 4cm/1½in in diameter.

6   Bake in the preheated oven for 10–12 minutes until golden. Remove from the oven and leave to cool for a few minutes, then transfer to a wire rack to cool.

STORAGE

Can be stored in an airtight container for up to 5 days.

* Health Benefits

Cacao is chocolate in its raw unadulterated form and because it is relatively unprocessed it contains higher levels of antioxidants and is an excellent source of magnesium. It is not uncommon to be deficient in magnesium, but the mineral is crucial for the heart and can reduce blood pressure as well as encourage a feeling of calm.

Food Facts per Biscuit

Calories 136kcal • **Total Carbs** 3.6g• **total sugar** 2g • **added sugar** 1.3g

(V) 🌿 🌾 🧀 🎲

Double-ginger Oat Cookies

You get a double helping of ginger in these delicious cookies: fresh root ginger and ground ginger both lend a wonderful flavour and aroma.

MAKES **12**   PREPARATION **15 minutes**   COOKING **17–20 minutes**

1 apple, cored and grated (unpeeled)

100g/3½oz/heaped ⅓ cup unsalted butter or coconut oil, plus extra
  for greasing

1 tbsp brown rice syrup, maple syrup or raw honey

2.5cm/1in piece fresh root ginger, peeled and grated

100g/3½oz/scant 1 cup wholemeal spelt flour

1 tsp baking powder

1 tsp ground ginger

pinch of salt

70g/2½oz/½ cup rolled jumbo oats

1   Preheat the oven to 180°C/350°F/Gas 4. Lightly grease 2 baking sheets.
    Put the apple in a small pan with 2 tablespoons water, cover with a
    lid, and cook gently, stirring regularly, for 10–12 minutes until tender.
    Remove from the heat and mash with the back of a fork or blend in a
    blender until puréed (you need about 85g/3oz purée). Leave to cool.

2   Melt the butter in a small saucepan with the syrup and grated ginger,
    then leave to cool slightly. Sift the flour (adding any bran left in the
    sieve), baking powder, ground ginger and pinch of salt into a mixing
    bowl and stir in the oats.

3   Add the melted butter and apple purée to the dry ingredients and
    stir to make a soft, chunky dough. Place heaped tablespoons of the
    cookie mixture onto the baking sheets and flatten the top of each
    cookie slightly.

4   Bake in the preheated oven for 15–18 minutes until light golden
    but still slightly soft. Remove from the oven and leave to cool for
    5 minutes, then transfer to a wire rack to cool completely.

STORAGE
Can be stored in an airtight container for up to 5 days.

* Health Benefits
   *Ginger is great for settling the stomach and relieving nausea. What's more,
   research indicates that ginger encourages the release of insulin in the body
   and increases the uptake of glucose in fat cells.*

Food Facts per Cookie
Calories 118kcal • **Total Carbs** 11.1g • **total sugar** 2.1g • **added sugar** 0.7g

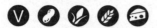

Walnut Shortbreads

These light, crumbly biscuits contain a minimum amount of sugar, but you would never know it. They are delicious topped with whipped cream and fresh strawberries or raspberries for a special dessert.

MAKES 15   PREPARATION **15 minutes**   COOKING **15–18 minutes**

115g/4oz/scant ½ cup chilled unsalted butter, diced, plus extra for greasing

150g/5½oz/scant 1½ cups wholemeal spelt flour, plus extra for dusting

30g/1oz/¼ cup oatmeal

1 tsp cinnamon

1 tsp baking powder

¼ tsp salt

2 tbsp xylitol

40g/1½oz/¼ cup walnuts, chopped

1 tbsp milk

1   Preheat the oven to 180°C/350°F/Gas 4. Lightly grease 2 baking sheets.

2   Sift the flour (adding any bran left in the sieve), oatmeal, cinnamon, baking powder and salt into a mixing bowl and stir in the xylitol. Rub in the butter with your fingertips until the mixture resembles fine breadcrumbs.

3   Stir in the walnuts, then the milk, then form the mixture into a soft dough with your hands.

4   Flour a work surface and rolling pin, then roll out the dough until 5mm/¼in thick. Using a 5cm/2in cutter, stamp out 15 biscuits, re-rolling the dough as necessary.

5   Place the biscuits on the baking sheets, then bake in the preheated oven for 15–18 minutes until golden. Remove from the oven and transfer to a wire rack to cool.

STORAGE
Can be stored in an airtight container for up to 5 days.

* Health Benefits

   Recent studies show that eating walnuts on a regular basis can reduce the risk of heart disease and lower levels of harmful LDL cholesterol in the body. Walnuts are also a good source of omega-3 fatty acids.

Food Facts per Biscuit

Calories 112kcal • **Total Carbs** 7.8g • **total sugar** 1.2g • **added sugar** 0g

Lemon & Ginger Cheesecake

The base of this cheesecake is made from oatcakes, nuts and seeds with a touch of ginger, while the light and lemony topping is reminiscent of that found on a baked New York cheesecake.

SERVES **12**   PREPARATION **25 minutes**   COOKING **45–55 minutes**

300g/10½oz/generous 1¼ cups low-fat cream cheese

200g/7oz/scant 1 cup half-fat crème fraîche

2 tsp vanilla extract

3 eggs, separated

1 tbsp brown rice syrup, maple syrup or raw honey

2 tbsp cornflour dissolved in 1 tbsp warm water

finely grated zest of 3 unwaxed lemons and juice of 2 lemons

3 tbsp xylitol

For the base:

60g/2¼oz/4 tbsp unsalted butter or coconut oil, melted, plus extra
   for greasing

120g/4½oz rough oatcakes

60g/2¼oz/scant ½ cup mixed nuts, such as cashews, Brazils and walnuts

2 tbsp sunflower seeds

2 tsp ground ginger

2 tbsp xylitol

1   First make the base. Preheat the oven to 160°C/315°F/Gas 3. Lightly grease a 20cm/8in springform cake tin/pan. Put the oatcakes in a food processor and process until they form a fine breadcrumb consistency.

2   Pour the crumbs into a mixing bowl. Put the nuts and seeds into the food processor and process until very finely chopped, then add to the bowl with the ground ginger, xylitol and melted butter. Stir until combined, then spoon into the prepared tin/pan and press firmly into an even layer to make a firm base.

3   To make the filling, put the cream cheese, crème fraîche, vanilla extract, egg yolks and syrup in a bowl and beat together. Add the dissolved cornflour, lemon zest and lemon juice and beat well.

4   Whisk the egg whites in a grease-free bowl until they form stiff peaks, then whisk in the xylitol. Using a metal spoon, fold the whites into the cream cheese mixture until they are well combined. Spoon the mixture into the cake tin/pan in an even layer.

5   Bake in the preheated oven for 45–55 minutes until the filling has set. Remove from the oven and leave to cool in the tin/pan.

STORAGE

Can be covered and stored in the refrigerator for up to 5 days.

* Health Benefits

Nuts and seeds often get a bad press due to their fat content, but remember that it is the healthier, unsaturated type of fat.

Food Facts per Portion

Calories 250kcal • **Total Carbs** 12.6g • **total sugar** 4.5g • **added sugar** 1.1g

Ⓥ ◉ ◉ ◉ ◉ ◉

Apple & Raspberry Flapjack Pie

Fruit crumble with a twist: this pie has a crisp oaty topping. Sweet apples are used instead of cooking apples, because they need much less added sugar to sweeten them. Make little pies in individual dishes rather than one large pie in a large dish, if you prefer.

SERVES 6 PREPARATION **15 minutes** COOKING **20–25 minutes**

3 sweet apples, quartered, cored, peeled and diced

squeeze of lemon juice

200g/7oz/1½ cups raspberries

2 tsp cinnamon

For the topping:

2 tbsp brown rice syrup, maple syrup or raw honey

90g/2¼oz unsalted butter or coconut oil

100g/3½oz/scant 1 cup rolled jumbo oats

3 tbsp chopped hazelnuts

2 tbsp chopped pecans

2 tbsp sunflower seeds

1 Preheat the oven to 180°C/350°F/Gas 4. Toss the apples in the lemon
   juice to prevent them browning, then place in a 20cm/8in ovenproof
   dish with 2 tablespoons water, the raspberries and cinnamon and stir
   well to combine.

2 To make the topping, heat the syrup and butter in a medium saucepan
   until the butter has melted. Remove from the heat and stir in the oats,
   hazelnuts, pecans and sunflower seeds.

3 Sprinkle the oat mixture over the top of the fruit. Bake in the
   preheated oven for 20–25 minutes until golden and beginning to crisp.
   Remove from the oven and serve warm.

STORAGE
Can be covered and stored in the refrigerator for up to 3 days.

* Health Benefits
*Raspberries are much lower in natural sugar than most other fruits and
are rich in vitamins A, C and E. They are also a good source of B vitamins,
which aid the metabolism of proteins, carbohydrates and fats in the body.*

Food Facts per Portion
Calories 325kcal • **Total Carbs** 25.5g • **total sugar** 10g • **added sugar** 4.5g

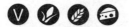

Black Forest Strudel

The star anise, cloves and cinnamon give a wonderful aroma, flavour and natural sweetness to this fruit strudel, which is packed with blackberries, blackcurrants, blueberries and apples. For convenience (and economy), use the bags of mixed frozen fruits that can be found in most large supermarkets. Serve with a spoonful of unsweetened coconut yogurt.

SERVES **6**   PREPARATION **15 minutes**   COOKING **35–40 minutes**

25g/1oz/2 tbsp unsalted butter or coconut oil, melted, plus
   extra for greasing
400g/14oz/2¼ cups frozen mixed black forest fruits,
   defrosted and drained
1 sweet apple, cored and grated (unpeeled)
1 star anise
3 cloves
1 heaped tsp ground cinnamon
2 tbsp xylitol or large pinch of stevia, to taste
2 tsp cornflour
9 sheets filo pastry, each about 30 × 18cm/12 × 7in

1   Preheat the oven to 190°C/375°F/Gas 5. Lightly grease a baking tray. Put the fruit in a saucepan with the star anise, cloves, cinnamon and xylitol. Stir and cook over a low heat for 3 minutes. Mix the cornflour with 1 tablespoon warm water and add to the pan. Cook, stirring occasionally, for another 3 minutes, then leave to cool.

2   Place a sheet of filo lengthways on the tray and brush lightly with some of the melted butter. Place a second sheet crossways over the first, so half of it overlaps, and another sheet next to it to make a 36 × 30cm/ 14 × 12in rectangle. Brush with more butter, then repeat this process twice more with the other 6 sheets.

3   Remove the star anise and cloves from the fruit, then spoon the mixture down the centre of the pastry, following the line of the first filo sheet, leaving a 2cm/¾in border. Carefully fold the filo over the fruit, tuck in the ends and then gently roll the parcel over so the seam is underneath.

4   Brush the top with the remaining butter and bake in the preheated oven for 30–35 minutes until golden and crisp. Remove from the oven and cut into slices before serving.

STORAGE

Can be stored in an airtight container in the refrigerator for up to 2 days. Reheat to crisp up the pastry.

* Health Benefits

Blackberries, blackcurrants and blueberries are a potent source of beneficial phytochemicals, anthocyanins and antioxidants.

Food Facts per Portion

Calories 117kcal • **Total Carbs** 13.3g • **total sugar** 6.5g • **added sugar** 0g

Ⓥ ◐ 🌿 🌾 🧀 🎲

Raspberry Cream Roulade

*A real treat of a pudding – this light "meringue" roulade is filled with
a rich and creamy vanilla coconut yogurt and fresh raspberries.*

SERVES **8**   PREPARATION **15 minutes**   COOKING **20–25 minutes**

unsalted butter or coconut oil, for greasing

4 large/extra-large egg whites

100g/3½oz/½ cup xylitol

40g/1½oz/⅓ cup self-raising flour

pinch of salt

For the filling:

125g/4½oz/¾ cup raspberries

125ml/4fl oz/½ cup 2% fat Greek yogurt

125ml/4fl oz/½ cup unsweetened coconut yogurt

1 tsp vanilla extract

2 tsp xylitol or pinch of stevia, to taste

1   Preheat the oven to 160°C/315°F/Gas 3. Line the base of a 20 × 30cm/
8 × 12in Swiss/jelly roll tin with parchment paper, then lightly grease the
sides of the tin and the paper. Whisk the egg whites in a large, grease-
free bowl until they form stiff peaks. Whisk in all but 1 teaspoon of the
xylitol, gradually sift in the flour and salt, then fold them in. Spoon the
mixture into the prepared tin and spread gently into an even layer.

2   Bake in the preheated oven for 20–25 minutes until golden and
    beginning to come away from the sides of the tin. Remove from the
    oven and leave to cool for a few minutes, then cover with a just-damp
    tea towel to prevent cracking when it is rolled up.

3   When the sponge has cooled, remove the tea towel. Lay a sheet of
    parchment paper on the work surface and sprinkle with the reserved
    xylitol. Turn the sponge out onto the paper and peel off the lining
    paper. Roll up the sponge carefully from the long side, wrapping the
    sugared paper inside, then leave to cool.

4   Put the raspberries in a mixing bowl with the yogurt, vanilla extract
    and xylitol. Stir gently until the ingredients have combined and
    the raspberries start to break down. Unroll the sponge, spread the
    raspberry cream over the top, then roll up and cut into slices.

STORAGE

Can be covered and stored in the refrigerator for up to 2 days.

* Health Benefits

*Xylitol is a low-calorie, crystallized sugar substitute. It is absorbed more slowly
than refined sugar so does not contribute to swings in blood-sugar levels.*

Food Facts per Portion

Calories 98kcal • **Total Carbs** 18.6g • **total sugar** 4.4g • **added sugar** 1g

Ⓥ 🥜 🌙 🌿 🌾 🎲

Blueberry Muffins

These muffins can be whipped up in a matter of minutes and make use of ground almonds and brown rice syrup in place of highly refined white flour and sugar.

MAKES **6**   PREPARATION **15 minutes**   COOKING **15 minutes**

3 tbsp olive oil, plus extra for greasing

2 eggs, lightly beaten

1 tsp vanilla extract

2 tbsp brown rice syrup, maple syrup or raw honey

100g/3½oz/scant 1 cup ground almonds

1 tsp baking powder

100g/3½oz/heaped ½ cup blueberries

1   Preheat the oven to 180°C/350°F/Gas 4. Lightly grease 6 holes of a deep muffin tin/pan. Whisk together the olive oil, eggs, vanilla extract and syrup in a mixing bowl.

2   Add the almonds, baking powder and blueberries and fold in gently
    without over-mixing, since this will make the muffins heavy.

3   Spoon the mixture into the muffin tin/pan and bake in the preheated
    oven for 15 minutes until risen and light golden. Remove the muffins
    from the oven and leave in the tin/pan for 5 minutes before turning out
    to cool on a wire rack.

STORAGE

Can be stored in an airtight container for up to 5 days.

* Health Benefits

*In addition to their cholesterol-lowering properties, almonds have an
ability to reduce the risk of heart disease, which has been partly attributed
to their high vitamin E content. The ground variety also makes a great
alternative to wheat flour in cakes and biscuits.*

Food Facts per Muffin

Calories 205kcal • **Total Carbs** 6.3g • **total sugar** 5.6g • **added sugar** 3.6g

Variation

In place of the blueberries, try using raspberries, dried cherries or
chopped dried apricots.

Carrot & Walnut Cake

Along with adding sweetness to a cake, sugar keeps it moist too: a role here that is partly taken on by the carrots. This is a delicious and simple cake to make. Lucuma, a South American fruit, makes a useful natural sweetener and is a good source of vitamins and minerals. Find it in health food stores and online.

SERVES **16**   PREPARATION **20 minutes**   COOKING **45 minutes**

unsalted butter or coconut oil, for greasing

125g/4½oz/generous 1 cup self-raising wholemeal flour

125g/4½oz/generous 1 cup self-raising flour

1 tbsp ground cinnamon

1 tbsp mixed spice/apple pie spice

2 tsp lucuma powder

100g/3½oz/scant ½ cup xylitol

300g/10½oz (about 3) carrots, peeled and finely grated

50g/1¾oz/½ cup chopped walnuts

200ml/7fl oz/generous ¾ cup coconut oil, melted

4 eggs

1–2 tbsp unsweetened almond milk (optional)

1   Preheat the oven to 180°C/350°F/Gas 4. Lightly grease and line the base of a 20cm/8in square cake tin.

2   Sift both types of flour (adding any bran left in the sieve), cinnamon and mixed spice/apple pie spice into a mixing bowl. Using a wooden spoon, stir in the lucuma powder, xylitol and carrots until combined. Next, stir in the walnuts.

3   Beat together the oil and eggs in a measuring jug, then pour the mixture into the mixing bowl and stir gently until all the ingredients are mixed together. Add the almond milk if the cake mixture seems too stiff; it should be of dropping consistency.

4   Pour the cake mixture into the prepared tin and smooth the top with the back of a spoon. Bake in the preheated oven for 40–45 minutes until risen and golden. Remove the cake from the oven and leave in the tin for 10 minutes, then turn it out to cool on a wire rack. Serve cut into squares.

STORAGE
Can be stored in an airtight tin or wrapped in foil for up to 5 days.

* Health Benefits
The antioxidant beta carotene (converted into vitamin A in the body) is found in plentiful amounts in carrots. A recent study also showed that carrots can help to protect against food poisoning.

Food Facts per Portion
Calories 230kcal • **Total Carbs** 18.2g • **total sugar** 5.9g • **added sugar** 0g

(V) (O) (V) (V) (OO) (O)

Banana Bread

A real family favourite, this bread makes a sustaining and nutritious teatime or coffee-break treat. Make sure you use ripe bananas, as they will give a delicious moistness and sweet flavour to this tea loaf.

SERVES **12**   PREPARATION **20 minutes**   COOKING **1 hour**

100g/3½oz/heaped ⅓ cup butter or coconut oil, plus extra
   for greasing
100g/3½oz/scant 1 cup plain/all-purpose flour
125g/4½oz/generous 1 cup plain/all-purpose wholemeal flour
1 tsp mixed spice/apple pie spice
1 heaped tsp baking powder
70g/2½oz/scant ½ cup unsulphured ready-to-eat dried apricots,
   roughly chopped
2 large/extra-large eggs, lightly beaten
2 tbsp brown rice syrup, maple syrup or raw honey
finely grated zest of 2 oranges and juice of 1 orange
3 ripe bananas, mashed

1   Preheat the oven to 180°C/350°F/Gas 4. Lightly grease and line the base
    of a 28 × 11 × 8cm/11¼ × 4¼ × 3¼in deep loaf tin/pan. Melt the butter
    in a small saucepan and leave to cool.

2   Sift both types of flour (adding any bran left in the sieve), mixed spice/
    apple pie spice and baking powder into a mixing bowl, then stir in the
    dried apricots.

3   Mix together the melted butter, eggs, syrup, orange juice and zest, then
    stir in the mashed bananas. Using a wooden spoon, gently stir the
    banana mixture into the dry ingredients – but don't over-mix or the
    cake will be heavy.

4   Pour the cake mixture into the prepared tin/pan and level the top, then
    bake in the preheated oven for 1 hour or until a skewer inserted into
    the centre of the cake comes out clean. Remove from the oven and
    leave in the tin for 10 minutes, then turn out onto a wire rack to cool.

STORAGE
Can be stored in an airtight container or wrapped in foil for up to 5 days.

* Health Benefits
*Bananas, when ripe, are a good way of adding natural sweetness to cakes
and biscuits. What's more, the fruit also provides beneficial amounts of
dietary fibre and minerals, especially potassium, which is important for the
cells, nerves and muscles. They are also rich in tryptophan, which is known
to lift the spirits and aid restful sleep.*

Food Facts per Portion
Calories 166kcal • **Total Carbs** 22.1g • **total sugar** 9.3g • **added sugar** 2.2g

Spiced Apple Cake

Apples lend a natural sweetness and moist texture to this simple cake, which is perfect as a teatime treat. The cake could also be served as a dessert with a dollop of fromage frais.

SERVES 12   PREPARATION **15 minutes**   COOKING **40 minutes**

125g/4¼oz/1 cup butter or coconut oil, melted, plus extra for greasing

3 apples (about 300g/10½oz), cored and grated (unpeeled)

115g/4oz/1 cup self-raising wholemeal flour

115g/4oz/1 cup self-raising flour

1 tbsp mixed spice/apple pie spice

1 tbsp ground cinnamon

80g/2¾oz/scant ½ cup xylitol

1 tbsp lucuma powder

2 eggs, lightly beaten

2–4 tbsp milk

1   Preheat the oven to 180°C/350°F/Gas 4. Lightly grease and line the base of a 20cm/8in springform cake tin.

2   Put the apples in a saucepan with 5 tablespoons water, cover with a lid, and cook gently, stirring regularly, for 10–12 minutes until tender. Remove from the heat and mash with the back of a fork or blend in a blender until puréed. Leave to cool.

3   Sift both types of flour (adding any bran left in the sieve), mixed spice/
    apple pie spice and cinnamon into a mixing bowl, then add the xylitol
    and lucuma. Stir the melted butter, eggs and enough milk into the dry
    ingredients to make a loose batter. Next, gently stir in the apples.

4   Tip the cake mixture into the prepared tin and level the top. Bake in
    the preheated oven for 35–40 minutes until risen and golden. Remove
    from the oven and leave to cool in the tin for 10 minutes, then transfer
    to a wire rack to cool.

STORAGE
Can be stored in an airtight container or wrapped in foil for up to 5 days.

* Health Benefits
Apples contain the trace mineral boron, which has been found to play an important role in maintaining mental alertness and concentration. Research also shows that boron may relieve the symptoms of arthritis, osteoporosis and candida.

Food Facts per Portion

Calories 182kcal • **Total Carbs** 21.1g • **total sugar** 2.6g • **added sugar** 0g

Variation
To use stevia instead of xylitol, add 1–3 tsp powdered stevia (depending on the brand and sweetness) and add 1 extra egg, 2 tbsp brown rice syrup, maple syrup or raw honey and 1 tsp baking powder.

Chocolate & Beetroot Brownies

These brownies make a wonderful treat with their moist "fudgy" texture and rich chocolate flavour. They're also gluten-free and so are suitable for those with a wheat allergy or intolerance.

SERVES **16**   PREPARATION **20 minutes**   COOKING **25–30 minutes**

100g/3½oz/heaped ⅓ cup unsalted butter or coconut oil,
   plus extra for greasing
115g/4oz dark/baking chocolate (75% cocoa solids), broken into squares
1 tsp vanilla extract
100g/3½oz/scant 1 cup ground almonds
80g/2¾oz/⅓ cup xylitol
1 tbsp brown rice syrup, maple syrup or raw honey
2 tbsp unsweetened cocoa powder
80g/2¾oz/½ cup Brazil nuts, roughly chopped
4 eggs, separated
175g/6oz cooked beetroot, patted dry and coarsely grated

1   Preheat the oven to 180°C/350°C/Gas 4. Grease and line the base of a 20cm/8in square tin/pan. Melt the butter and chocolate in a heatproof bowl placed over a saucepan of gently simmering water, making sure the bottom of the bowl does not touch the water.

2   Remove the bowl from the heat, stir, then leave to cool slightly. Stir in
    the vanilla extract, ground almonds, xylitol, syrup, cocoa powder and
    Brazil nuts and mix well until combined. Beat the egg yolks lightly,
    then stir them into the chocolate mixture with the beetroot.

3   Whisk the egg whites in a large, grease-free bowl until they form stiff
    peaks. Using a metal spoon, stir a spoonful of the whites into the
    chocolate mixture to slacken it, then fold in the remaining egg whites
    until they are well combined.

4   Spoon the mixture into the prepared tin and bake in the preheated
    oven for 20–25 minutes until risen and firm on top but still slightly
    gooey in the centre. Remove from the oven and leave to cool in the tin,
    then turn out, remove the baking parchment and cut into 16 squares.

STORAGE
Can be stored in an airtight container for up to 5 days.

* Health Benefits
*Brazil nuts are particularly rich in the mood-enhancing mineral selenium.
A single nut a day will ensure that you are not deficient in this mineral.*

Food Facts per Brownie

Calories 206kcal • **Total Carbs** 11.4g • **total sugar** 3.9g • **added sugar** 1g

Ⓥ ⓞ 🌿 🌾 🧀 🎲

Chocolate & Orange Cake

Treat yourself to this rich, intensely chocolatey cake-cum-dessert.
Serve with a good spoonful of fromage frais.

SERVES 12   PREPARATION **15 minutes**   COOKING **25–30 minutes**

50g/1¾oz/3 tbsp butter or coconut oil, plus extra for greasing
60g/2¼oz dark/baking chocolate (75% cocoa solids), broken intro squares
3 eggs, separated
4 tbsp xylitol
finely grated zest of 2 oranges and juice of 1 orange
70g/2½oz/scant ⅔ cup self-raising flour
2 tbsp unsweetened cocoa powder

1   Preheat the oven to 150°C/300°F/Gas 2. Lightly grease and line the base of a 20cm/8in springform cake tin.

2   Melt the butter and chocolate in a heatproof bowl placed over a saucepan of gently simmering water, making sure the bottom of the bowl does not touch the water. Stir occasionally until the chocolate and butter have melted, then remove from the heat.

3   Whisk the egg yolks with the xylitol in a mixing bowl until pale, then stir in the chocolate mixture followed by the orange juice and zest. Sift the flour and cocoa powder into the chocolate mixture and fold in using a wooden spoon.

4   Whisk the egg whites in a large, grease-free mixing bowl until they form stiff peaks. Using a metal spoon, stir a spoonful of the whites into the chocolate mixture to slacken it, then fold in the remaining egg whites until they are well combined.

5   Spoon the mixture into the prepared cake tin, then bake in the preheated oven for 20–25 minutes until risen. Remove from the oven and leave in the tin for 10 minutes, then turn out to cool on a wire rack.

STORAGE
Can be stored in an airtight container for up to 5 days.

* Health Benefits
  Make sure you buy a good-quality dark/baking chocolate, at least 75 per cent cocoa solids, since its sugar content should be lower than other types of dark/baking chocolate with a reduced percentage of cocoa.

Food Facts per Portion
Calories 120kcal • **Total Carbs** 12.5g • **total sugar** 4.1g • **added sugar** 0.5g

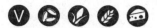

Seeded Oatcakes

Serve these light oatcakes plain or topped with humous, pâté or low-fat cream cheese for a more substantial snack.

MAKES 24   PREPARATION 20 **minutes**   COOKING 10 **minutes**

sunflower oil, for greasing

175g/6oz/1½ cups wholemeal spelt flour, plus extra for dusting

100g/3½oz/scant 1 cup medium oatmeal

2 tsp baking powder

¼ tsp salt

100g/3½oz/heaped ⅓ cup chilled unsalted butter, diced

2 tsp xylitol

2 tbsp sunflower seeds

4 tbsp semi-skimmed milk

1   Preheat the oven to 200°C/400°F/Gas 6. Lightly grease 2 baking sheets. Sift the flour (adding any bran left in the sieve), oatmeal, baking powder and salt into a mixing bowl.

2   Add the butter and rub it into the flour mixture using your fingertips until the mixture resembles breadcrumbs, then stir in the xylitol and sunflower seeds. Pour in the milk and mix with a fork, and then your hands, to make a dough.

3 Turn the dough out on to a lightly floured work surface and knead briefly until smooth. Using a floured rolling pin, roll out the dough into a rectangle about 5mm/¼in thick. Trim the edges and cut into about 24 squares, re-rolling any trimmings as necessary.

4 Place the oatcakes on the baking sheets and prick the tops with a fork. Bake in the preheated oven for 10 minutes until light golden, swapping the trays halfway, if necessary. Remove from the oven and transfer to a wire rack to cool.

STORAGE

Can be stored in an airtight container for up to 5 days.

* Health Benefits

Oats and wholemeal flour provide both soluble and insoluble fibre. The former, found in most fruits, oats and pulses, helps to regulate levels of cholesterol and glucose in the body. Insoluble fibre, found in whole grains, fruit and vegetables, keeps the bowels regular.

Food Facts per Oatcake

Calories 82kcal • **Total Carbs** 8.1g • **total sugar** 0.7g • **added sugar** 0g

Cheese & Rosemary Scones

The secret to successful sweet or savoury scones is to avoid over-mixing the dough; treat it kindly and you'll be rewarded with light and fluffy scones. The cheese adds valuable protein, while the flaxseeds provide omega-3 fatty acids. The scones are best eaten when still warm.

MAKES **10**   PREPARATION **10 minutes**   COOKING **15 minutes**

200g/7oz/1⅓ cups self-raising wholemeal spelt flour, plus extra for dusting.
¼ tsp salt
2 tsp ground flaxseeds
1 tbsp chopped rosemary
½ tsp mustard powder
125g/4½oz half-fat strong Cheddar cheese, grated
50g/1¾oz unsalted butter, cubed
100ml/3½fl oz/scant ½ cup semi-skimmed milk, plus extra for brushing

1   Preheat the oven to 220°C/425°F/Gas 7. Line a baking sheet with parchment paper.

2   Sift the flour into a mixing bowl, adding any bran left in the sieve, and stir in the salt, flaxseeds, rosemary, mustard powder and 100g/3½oz of the Cheddar. Using your fingertips, rub in the butter until you have a coarse crumb texture. Gradually, add the milk and bring the dough together with your hands.

3   Roll the dough out on a lightly floured work surface until about 2cm/¾in thick. Using a 4.5cm/1¾in cutter, stamp out 10 scones. Brush the top of each scone with milk and sprinkle with the remaining Cheddar. Bake for 12–15 minutes until risen and golden. Leave to cool slightly on a wire rack. Serve warm or leave to cool.

STORAGE
Can be stored in an airtight container for up to 3 days.

* Health Benefits
Studies show that flaxseeds may help to protect against breast cancer, diabetes and heart disease. High-fibre flaxseeds are an excellent plant source of omega-3 fatty acids and also provide lignans, which have antioxidant properties.

Food Facts per Scone
Calories 139kcal • **Total Carbs** 1.7g • **total sugar** 0.8g • **added sugar** 0g

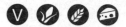

Spelt Soda Bread

If you haven't made bread before, soda bread is the perfect place to start. It's quick to make because it doesn't need rising, but the end result is delicious – especially when still warm.

MAKES **1 loaf**   PREPARATION **15 minutes**   COOKING **40 minutes**

450g/1lb/4 cups wholemeal spelt flour, plus extra for dusting
1 tsp baking soda
1 tsp salt
275ml/9½fl oz/generous 1 cup buttermilk
2 tbsp natural low-fat bio yogurt

1   Preheat the oven to 200°C/400°F/Gas 6. Dust a large baking sheet with flour.

2   Sift the flour (adding any bran left in the sieve), baking soda and salt into a mixing bowl and make a well in the centre. Pour in the buttermilk and yogurt, then gently mix with outstretched fingers to make a soft, slightly sticky dough.

3 Turn the dough out on to a lightly floured work surface and gently form into a smooth ball – don't over-knead or the bread will be heavy. Press the top of the dough down slightly with the palm of your hand.

4 Cut a deep cross into the dough, and, if you're into Irish folklore, don't forget to prick each quarter so the fairies in the dough can get out! Sift a little flour over the top and bake in the preheated oven for 35–40 minutes until risen and golden. Remove from the oven and transfer to a wire rack to cool.

STORAGE
Can be stored in an airtight container or wrapped in foil for up to 5 days.

* Health Benefits
Low-fat yogurt is a good source of protein, zinc, B vitamins and bone-building calcium. It also provides beneficial bacteria that can help to maintain a healthy digestive system.

Food Facts per Slice (loaf makes 12)
Calories 128kcal • **Total Carbs** 23.8g • **total sugar** 2.3g • **added sugar** 0g

Menu Plans

WHEAT & GLUTEN-FREE 5-DAY MENU

For those people who are allergic to or intolerant of wheat and gluten, this menu is easy-to-follow, balanced and, what's more, low in sugar. It may also be necessary to monitor your intake of carbohydrate foods, especially if diabetic, and this menu will allow you to do this.

Day 1

BREAKFAST: Chia Breakfast Pudding (see page 50)

LUNCH: Chinese Egg & Prawn Rice (see page 100)

DINNER: Chicken with Gazpacho Salsa (see page 142)

Day 2

BREAKFAST: On-the-day Muesli (see page 46)

LUNCH: Asparagus, Courgette & Chive Omelette (see page 94)

DINNER: Beef & Lentil Curry (see page 146)

Day 3

BREAKFAST: More-fish-than-rice Kedgeree (see page 64)

LUNCH: Warm Greek Salad of Beans, Basil & Feta (see page 84)

DINNER: Marinated Lamb with Chickpea Mash (see page 154)

Day 4

BREAKFAST: Fig & Vanilla Breakfast Yogurt (see page 42)

LUNCH: Bacon, Lentil & Pepper Salad (see page 112)

DINNER: Lemon & Spinach Lentils with Egg (see page 120)

Day 5

BREAKFAST: Cheese & Tomato Soufflés (see page 56)

LUNCH: Turkey & Apple Salad (see page 110)

DINNER: Spice-crusted Salmon with Cucumber Salad (see page 126)

VEGETARIAN 5-DAY MENU

This menu is designed to provide all the nutrients required when following a low-sugar, vegetarian diet, which is free from meat, poultry and seafood.

Day 1

BREAKFAST: Cottage Cheese Pancakes (see page 58)

LUNCH: Tomato & Lentil Soup (see page 82)

DINNER: Vegetarian Chilli in Tortilla Baskets (see page 122)

Day 2

BREAKFAST: Cinnamon Porridge with Pear (see page 48)

LUNCH: Warm Greek Salad of Beans, Basil & Feta (see page 84)

DINNER: Masoor Dahl (see page 124)

Day 3

BREAKFAST: Fig & Vanilla Breakfast Yogurt (see page 42)

LUNCH: Avocado & Tomato Bruschetta (see page 88)

DINNER: Lemon & Spinach Lentils with Egg (see page 120)

Day 4

BREAKFAST: Cheese & Tomato Soufflés (see page 56)

LUNCH: Red Quinoa Tabbouleh (see page 86)

DINNER: Ribollita (see page 118)

Day 5

BREAKFAST: Fruity French Toast (see page 52)

LUNCH: Spicy Tofu Cakes with Dipping Sauce (see page 90)

DINNER: Huevos Rancheros (see page 92)

VEGAN 5-DAY MENU

This menu avoids any foods derived from animals, including meat, fish, poultry, eggs, dairy and honey. In some cases, recipes have been adapted to suit a vegan diet; use almond, soya, rice or oat milk, yogurt and cheese if appropriate.

Day 1
BREAKFAST: Avocado & Coconut Smoothie (see page 36)
LUNCH: Red Quinoa Tabbouleh (see page 86) – omit halloumi
DINNER: Vegetarian Chilli in Tortilla Baskets (see page 122) – omit sour cream

Day 2
BREAKFAST: Blueberry & Almond Bircher Muesli (see page 44)
LUNCH: Avocado & Tomato Bruschetta (see page 88)
DINNER: Masoor Dahl (see page 124)

Day 3
BREAKFAST: Home-made Baked Beans (see page 60)
LUNCH: Spicy Tofu Cakes (see page 90) – omit dip
DINNER: Ribollita (see page 118)

Day 4
BREAKFAST: Chia Breakfast Pudding (see page 50)
LUNCH: Tomato & Lentil Soup (see page 82)
DINNER: Huevos Rancheros (see page 92) – omit eggs and top with vegan cheese alternative and toasted cashews

Day 5
BREAKFAST: Cinnamon Porridge with Pear (see page 48)
LUNCH: Warm Greek Salad of Beans, Basil & Feta (see page 84) – vegan cheese
DINNER: Pasta Puttanesca (see page 98) – omit anchovies and sprinkle with pine nuts

NUT-FREE 5-DAY MENU

Allergies to nuts and seeds are becoming increasingly common, and, as the symptoms can be life-threatening, it is essential to take every precaution to avoid contact with nuts, seeds and by-products. Always check food labels.

Day 1
BREAKFAST: Banana Griddle Cakes (see page 184)
LUNCH: Salmon & Onion Frittata (see page 104)
DINNER: Moroccan Chicken Pilaf (see page 138)

Day 2
BREAKFAST: Sardines & Tomato on Toast (see page 66) – use unseeded bread
LUNCH: Turkey & Apple Salad (see page 110)
DINNER: Lemon & Spinach Lentils with Egg (see page 120)

Day 3
BREAKFAST: Fruity French Toast (see page 52) – use unseeded bread
LUNCH: Chinese Egg & Prawn Rice (see page 100)
DINNER: Ham & Barley Broth (see page 150)

Day 4
BREAKFAST: Home-made Baked Beans (see page 60)
LUNCH: Spiced Chicken with Lime Guacamole (see page 106)
DINNER: Seafood Hotpot with Rouille (see page 130)

Day 5
BREAKFAST: More-fish-than-rice Kedgeree (see page 64)
LUNCH: Beef & Broccoli Stir-fry (see page 114)
DINNER: Vegetarian Chilli in Tortilla Baskets (see page 122)

Index

Notes